Maintenance and repair of laboratory, diagnostic imaging, and hospital equipment

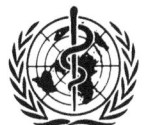

World Health Organization
Geneva
1994

WHO Library Cataloguing in Publication Data

Maintenance and repair of laboratory, diagnostic imaging, and hospital equipment.

1. Diagnostic imaging   2. Equipment & supplies, Hospital   3. Maintenance

ISBN 92 4 154463 5   (NLM Classification: WX 147)

The World Health Organization welcomes requests for permission to reproduce or translate its publications, in part or in full. Applications and enquiries should be addressed to the Office of Publications, World Health Organization, Geneva, Switzerland, which will be glad to provide the latest information on any changes made to the text, plans for new editions, and reprints and translations already available.

© World Health Organization 1994

Publications of the World Health Organization enjoy copyright protection in accordance with the provisions of Protocol 2 of the Universal Copyright Convention. All rights reserved.

The designations employed and the presentation of the material in this publication do not imply the expression of any opinion whatsoever on the part of the Secretariat of the World Health Organization concerning the legal status of any country, territory, city or area or of its authorities, or concerning the delimitation of its frontiers or boundaries.

The mention of specific companies or of certain manufacturers' products does not imply that they are endorsed or recommended by the World Health Organization in preference to others of a similar nature that are not mentioned. Errors and omissions excepted, the names of proprietary products are distinguished by initial capital letters.

TYPESET IN INDIA
PRINTED IN FINLAND

93/9652-Macmillan/Vammalan-8000

Contents

Preface	v
Acknowledgements	vi
1. Introduction	**1**
2. Laboratory equipment	**3**
Autoclaves, ovens, incubators, and water-baths	3
Balances	8
Batteries	13
Cell counters	20
Centrifuges	22
Electrode equipment	26
Flame photometers	29
Gas cylinders and gases	33
Microscopes	38
Photometers	41
Pipettes, autopipettes, and dispensers	48
Refrigerators	52
Water purification systems	56
3. Diagnostic equipment	**61**
Blood pressure machines (sphygmomanometers)	61
Ophthalmoscopes and otoscopes	64
Laryngoscopes	65
Stethoscopes	67
Electrocardiograph machines and cardiac monitors	67
4. Anaesthetic and resuscitation equipment	**70**
Breathing machines	70
Infant incubators	72
Oxygen entrainment systems	73
Systems for continuous-flow anaesthesia	75
Vaporizers	79
Testing anaesthetic machines, ventilators and related equipment	93
5. Operation room equipment	**101**
Antistatic equipment and apparatus	101

Operating table ... 102
Suction apparatus ... 103
Surgical diathermy machine ... 105

6. Ultrasound equipment ... 108
Physical principles ... 108
The scanner ... 110
Scanning probes ... 111
Artefacts ... 112
The Doppler effect ... 112
Recording ... 113
Maintenance and repair ... 113
Specification of the scanner ... 119

7. X-ray diagnostic equipment ... 121
The production and use of X-rays ... 121
Components of the X-ray system ... 121
Maintenance and repair in the X-ray department ... 124
Before sending for the service engineer ... 133
General rules ... 134
Battery-powered generators ... 135

Selected further reading ... 136
Annex 1. The WHO Basic Radiological System (WHO-BRS) ... 137
Annex 2. Set of tools, instruments and machinery for a maintenance unit in a district hospital ... 145
Annex 3. Basic laboratory equipment ... 148
Annex 4. Physical units ... 149
Annex 5. Some common disinfectants, their dilutions for use, properties, and potential applications ... 150
Annex 6. Checklists for anaesthetic apparatus ... 151
Index ... 153

Preface

In any country, developed or developing, the majority of faults affecting laboratory and hospital equipment can be avoided if the user has a clear understanding of its operation. A lack of understanding of the construction and function of such equipment increases the degree of misuse and risk of damage and, in some cases, the danger to the patient.

Evidently, many of the laboratory, diagnostic imaging and hospital instruments currently in use are sophisticated and must be serviced by specialists in case of major breakdown. However, in many cases, breakdown can be avoided if certain basic rules of prevention are followed. Unfortunately, there are no textbooks and surprisingly little written information on the maintenance of basic laboratory, imaging and hospital equipment. Laboratories and hospitals in developing countries suffer particularly from the fact that much equipment is imported, while adequate information on maintenance and repair is rarely provided by the supplier.

This manual seeks to remedy the situation by providing practical guidance on the maintenance and repair of a range of laboratory and hospital equipment. The information it contains will be invaluable to staff responsible for ensuring proper care of such equipment during daily use, as well as to those conducting training programmes.

The views expressed in this manual are those of the individual contributors. Comments on the usefulness of this manual, and suggestions for improvements in future editions will be welcome, and should be addressed to Health Laboratory Technology and Blood Safety, World Health Organization, 1211 Geneva 27, Switzerland.

Acknowledgements

This handbook has been prepared as a collaborative activity with contributions from the following:

Dr B. Breyer, Gynaecological Cancer Centre, Zagreb, Croatia;
Dr G. Gomez-Crespo, Segny, France;
Dr G. P. Hanson, Radiation Medicine, WHO, Geneva, Switzerland;
Dr C.-C. Heuck, Health Laboratory Technology and Blood Safety, WHO, Geneva, Switzerland;
Dr P. E. S. Palmer, Davis, CA, USA;
Mr A. Reich, Solenco, Monheim, Germany;
Mr M. Snook, Clinical Research Centre, Harrow, Middlesex, England;
Mr P. Vogt, Leysin, Switzerland;
Dr V. Volodin, Radiation Medicine, WHO, Geneva, Switzerland;
Dr A. E. O. Wasunna, Clinical Technology, WHO, Geneva, Switzerland;
Dr H. G. J. Worth, King's Mill Hospital, Sutton-in-Ashfield, Nottinghamshire, England;
Mr M. Yeats, Plymouth Hospitals, Plymouth, Devonshire, England.

The valuable suggestions of the following people are also gratefully acknowledged:

Mr V. Duenkel, Dar es Salaam, United Republic of Tanzania;
Mr R. Milton, St Paul's Hospital, Vancouver, Canada;
Mr K. O. Stross, Sipa Electronics, Schwabstadt, Germany.

Thanks are due to Mr J. Huys, Renkum, Netherlands for providing the illustrations for Figs 2.1 and 3.1.

1. Introduction

The maintenance of medical equipment is essential to ensure that it functions correctly and efficiently and ultimately to ensure proper clinical management of the patient. It is, therefore, important that adequate standards of maintenance are achieved. Yet, in some countries more than 60% of biomedical equipment is not used because of lack of facilities for maintenance and repair. These problems have no simple solution, and their implications are far wider than those associated with the maintenance of an individual piece of equipment.

Maintenance of equipment may be carried out by laboratory and hospital personnel employed to operate the instrument, by service personnel employed within a hospital service department, by technicians with special knowledge of a particular instrument, or by engineers with specialist expertise. This manual provides practical guidelines for use in health care institutions that do not have technicians or engineers with specialist expertise. It does not cover the more sophisticated equipment found in large hospitals. It is anticipated that, for these items, reference will have to be made to the manufacturer for assistance.

Fundamental training is essential for the operators of equipment and for the hospital maintenance staff so that the hospital may become nearly self-sufficient and able to keep its equipment in good working order. Good maintenance and servicing should be carried out as a partnership between the hospital and the manufacturer. Inevitably, however, the smaller the input by the manufacturer, the greater must be the input by the hospital. In many countries the manufacturers' presence, or that of their agents, is minimal and so also is their support. The level of support should be ascertained and taken into account during the process of instrument selection and purchase.

The aims of maintenance are to ensure that equipment attains the standard performance characteristics set by the hospital, the manufacturer's specification, and the clinical requirements. It should be carried out on a preventive basis rather than after a breakdown. A major breakdown is a sign that the maintenance and servicing programmes have failed.

While the selection and purchase of equipment are not directly relevant to the theme of this manual, they need to be mentioned briefly. The selection of appropriate equipment is essential if it is to carry out effectively the job for which it is required. This must take into account not only the current but also the projected workloads.

Some manufacturers offer contracts to lend equipment—even free of charge—but often the user has to agree to use, for example, reagents produced and sold by the same company. Quite often, their cost, in the long term, far exceeds the cost of purchasing other equipment and reagents. However, the cost of the reagents can be spread over a longer period of time.

When the final decision is made, the problems of installation must also be considered. The electrical supply must be compatible with the requirements of the instrument, including the necessary stability. Other necessary services must be available; for example gas and water supplies must be available in appropriate quantity and quality. The operating environment must be suitable. Temperature and humidity control must be available, if necessary. The level of lighting must be adequate, and there must be sufficient working space. If the equipment is bulky, as in the case of X-ray equipment and some laboratory analysers, there must be facilities for moving the instrument to its working area. Stairways, elevators and doorways must be wide enough, and appropriate lifting gear must be available.

The costs of acquiring and using any piece of equipment may be divided into two categories, capital costs and running costs. The capital cost is recognized at the time of purchase, but the running costs are frequently not fully appreciated. This may result in inefficient use or, in extreme cases, total abandonment of the machine. Running costs must therefore be determined prior to purchase; they are of four main types:
— maintenance,
— manpower,
— services,
— consumables.

The cost of maintenance carried out by the manufacturer will vary from country to country. The annual cost of a comprehensive service contract may be as high as 15% of the current capital cost of the equipment. This may not be the cheapest form of maintenance, but, if the manufacturer's commitment is high, it is probably the most effective and is the most easily costed.

Manpower costs must include those of the operator and the personnel of the supporting services (excluding maintenance, which is considered above). Costs must include not only the salary, but all the costs of employment, such as insurance, employer's contribution to pension schemes, and other costs or taxes, as appropriate.

Services must include the cost of electricity, water, gases, and any other similar supplies that are required and represent a significant sum.

The day-to-day running costs of all materials must be included under the heading of consumables. For laboratory analysers, this would include reagents, plastics, calibrating and control materials, etc., and for X-ray machines, film, contrast media, chemicals for development, etc.

Whereas it is important to know what the overall running cost of each piece of equipment is, when budgeting for replacement equipment, it may be more important to know whether the new instrument will be more or less expensive, overall, than the one it is replacing.

Selection, purchase, and installation of equipment must be primarily the responsibility of the head of the department and his or her staff. In making such decisions, both the capital and running costs must be taken into account. When choosing equipment, account should be taken of the availability of spares and the supplier's willingness to train the hospital staff appropriately. Unfortunately, it is only too frequent that equipment has to be abandoned because its running costs have not been budgeted for. Often purchasing decisions are made outside the laboratory, for political or other non-specific reasons, and this contributes to the numerous pieces of medical and paramedical equipment that are not used effectively in many countries.

2. Laboratory equipment

The choice of laboratory equipment must take into account national regulations and the technical premises that determine the requirements for its appropriate use. The more complex an instrument is, the more the user will depend on the support of a supplier for maintenance; it is therefore pertinent to foresee the magnitude of the costs that may be involved in its use. Quite often, the costs for use and maintenance of an instrument will exceed the costs of purchase.

It is also important to foresee the problems that may arise in case of failure of the instrument. Sometimes it may be advisable to purchase an instrument from a company that offers a guaranteed service, instead of another, perhaps cheaper, instrument for which a local maintenance service is not available.

The operating manual describing the function, installation, and use of an instrument should be provided free by the supplier and read by the user prior to any purchase. This avoids any subsequent misunderstanding. For example, it should be assured that an adequate power supply, as recommended for the instrument, is available locally, otherwise the purchase may be useless, or the cost of adaptation will increase the effective purchase price considerably.

Autoclaves, ovens, incubators, and water-baths

Autoclaves, hot-air ovens, incubators, and water-baths are devices for heating air or water. The heat is usually generated by an electrical module, but in some instruments heat is generated by fire, or there may be a heat-storage block, such as a separate water reservoir in solar systems or a metal block controlled by a thermostat.

Autoclaves

Autoclaves generate steam from water at a temperature above 100 °C in a closed chamber (Fig. 2.1). At these temperatures, the steam is above atmospheric pressure, and the conditions are optimal for the sterilization of laboratory equipment, medical devices, and media used for microbial culture. Bacteria cannot survive in such an environment, but viruses are not necessarily killed. The temperature can be kept 30–40 °C lower than in dry-air ovens, so that temperature-sensitive materials can also be sterilized. However, autoclaves need careful handling and must be inspected regularly; they can be dangerous and cause serious injury if steam accidently escapes from the equipment.

Two types of autoclave are available. The non-jacketed autoclave, which exists in vertical and horizontal versions, is simpler and has some practical disadvantages, but it is cheaper than a steam-jacketed autoclave with automatic air and condenser discharge.

Sterilization of porous materials, like laundry and bandages, is more difficult, since the air in these materials must be replaced by steam. This replacement is improved by evacuating the closed chamber of the autoclave containing the materials to be sterilized. With modern autoclaves, the chamber can be repeatedly evacuated so that the pressure in the chamber falls to 5.5 kPa. The chamber is then heated to evaporate water for sterilization.

Fig. 2.1. A: Non-jacketed autoclave. B: Steam-jacketed autoclave.

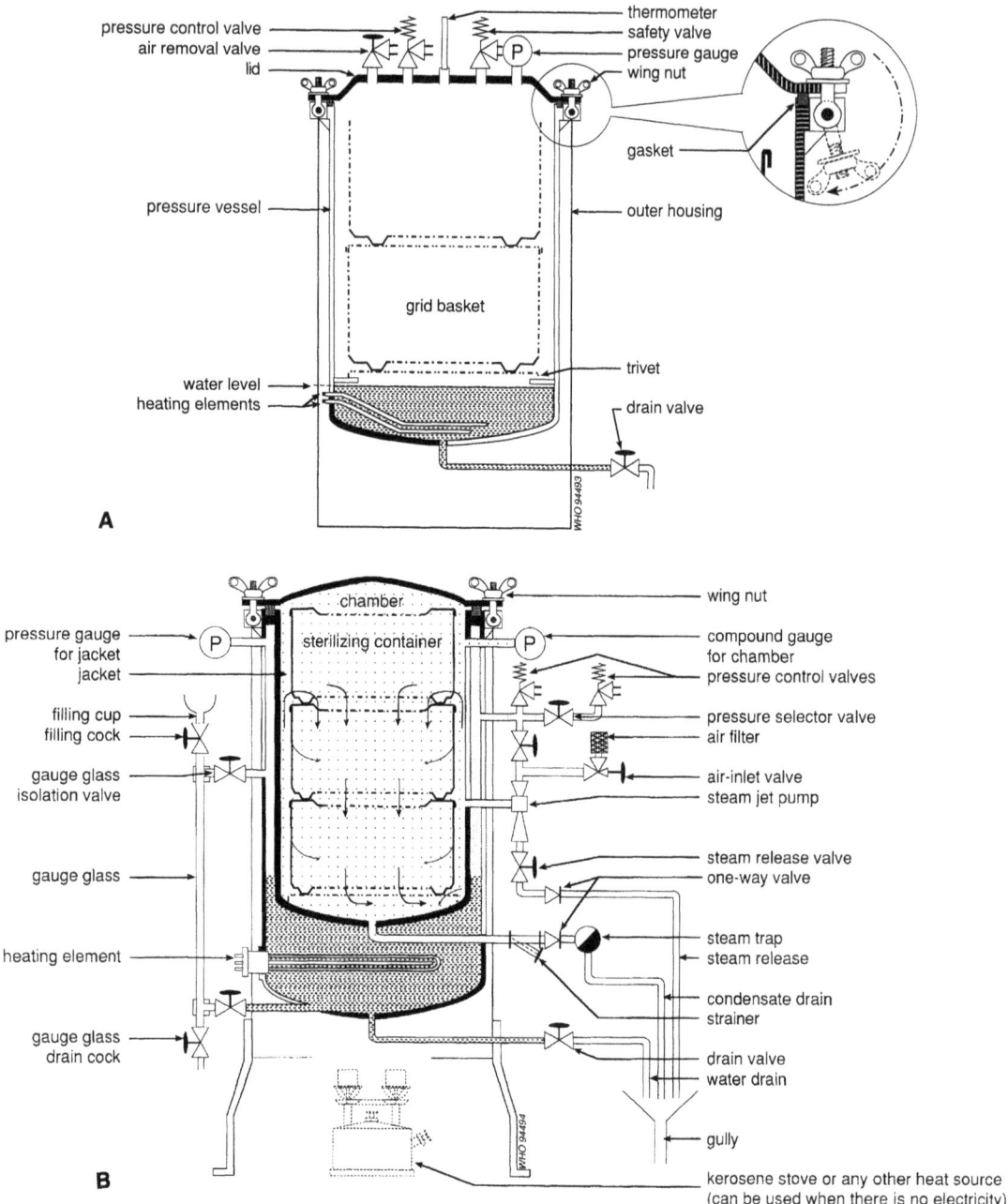

The main factors influencing steam sterilization are:

— saturated steam,
— temperature, and
— time.

The materials can be exposed to steam in a single heat cycle. However, this method of sterilization is less effective than intermittent exposure in three cycles over three days, which may kill all vegetative forms of sporulating microbes.[1] The cycle conditions may be shortened by increasing the pressure, and hence the temperature of the steam (Fig. 2.2). As with hot-air sterilization, effective steam

---

[1] In hospital microbiology, spores are defined as cells of microorganisms that withstand heating to 75 °C for 20 mins.

Fig. 2.2. Relation between steam pressure and temperature at constant volume.

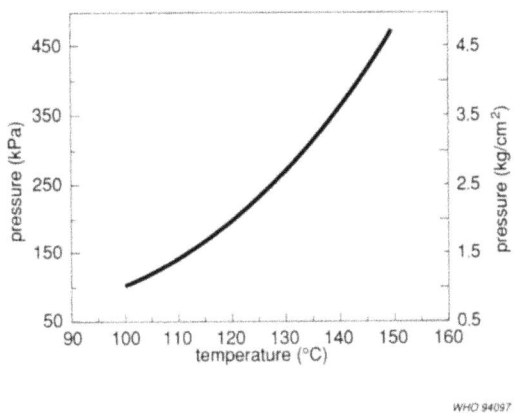

Fig. 2.3. Temperature variation during autoclave sterilization.

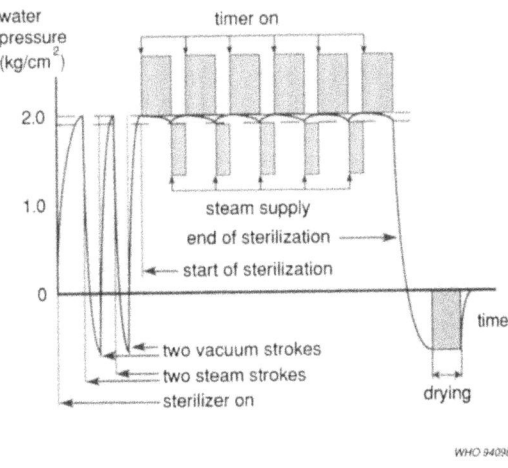

sterilization starts when the autoclave has reached the appropriate temperature (Fig. 2.3).

Suitable temperature and pressure regimes for operating autoclaves are shown in Table 2.1.

Table 2.1. Operating regimes for autoclaves

Sterilizing temperature (°C)	Appropriate pressure (kPa)	Minimum holding time (min)	Overall time (min)
115	75	30	50
122	115	15	40
128	150	10	30
136	225	3	20

Use of autoclaves

1. Prepare the material for autoclaving with indicator paper.
2. Fill the bottom of the autoclave with demineralized water, up to the support.
3. Place the material to be sterilized in the autoclave, close the lid and make sure that the rubber washer is in its groove. Screw down the clamps firmly.
4. Open the air outlet valve.
5. Turn on the heating (electric element, gas, burner, kerosene stove). Do not leave the autoclave unattended.
6. Close the outlet valve when a constant jet of steam issues from it. Reduce the heat supply so that it does not heat too quickly.
7. Once the expected temperature is reached, reduce the heating to maintain the temperature.
8. Do not touch the drainage tap or the outlet or safety valve while heating under pressure.
9. When the required time is up, turn off the heating completely.
10. When the temperature falls below 100°C, open the outlet valve slowly. Do not leave the outlet valve unopened for too long.
11. Never unscrew the lid clamps and open the lid until the hissing sound has stopped.
12. Leave the sterilized material to cool before removing it from the autoclave.
13. Check whether the autoclave tape (used for packaging of the material to be sterilized) has turned black and the covering paper has turned brown (not yellow or black).

Periodic inspection and cleaning

- Door gaskets should be kept clean and regularly checked for cracks and pitting due to deterioration.
- Door clamps and door locks should be checked for proper operation, and lubricated with high-temperature grease. The proper operation of the pressure locking device should be determined.
- Valve discs and seats must be inspected for signs of wear or cutting.
- Pressure gauges and thermometers should be checked periodically against a known standard.
- Adequate functioning of autoclaves should be checked weekly by the use of a biological (spore suspension) or chemical indicator. For biological testing, WHO recommends the use of *Bacillus stearothermophilus* ATCC 1953. For thermal control, commercially available chemical test strips that check the time and temperature exposure can be used.
- The function of manometers must be checked every 3 months.

Hot-air ovens

Hot-air ovens are used mainly for drying laboratory equipment and surgical devices in dry air. There are two types of hot-air oven, with and without internal circulation of dry air. Only small hot-air ovens can work without internal air circulation. Sterilization in dry air is less effective than steam sterilization, despite the higher temperatures applied (Table 2.2).

Although bacteria are killed at the higher temperatures, some spores can survive; also bacterial endotoxins are only partially inactivated. The temperature must be monitored in at least two areas of the sterilization chamber—preferably areas where the conditions for sterilization are most difficult to achieve. It is important to remember that the timing of sterilization should begin when the air in the oven has reached the required temperature (Fig. 2.4).

Table 2.2. Dry air sterilization in a hot-air oven

Temperature (°C)	Time (min)
160	180
170	120
180	30

Fig. 2.4. Temperature variation during hot air sterilization.

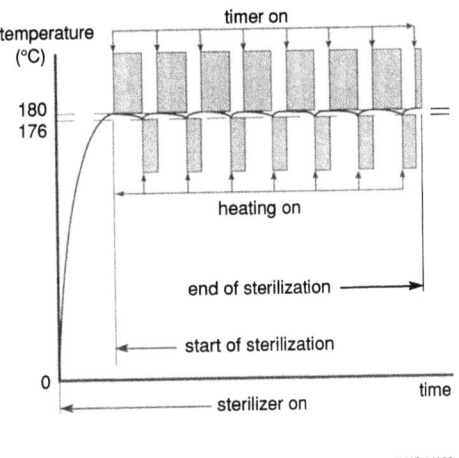

Use of hot-air ovens

1. Set the thermostat to the required temperature.
2. If there is a fan, check that it is working.
3. Allow to continue heating for the appropriate time after the temperature reaches the pre-set value.
4. Switch off the heating when time is up.
5. Wait until the temperature falls to 40 °C before opening the door.

Incubators

Incubators are used mainly for bacterial culture, but have additional uses within the laboratory. The incubator must maintain a constant temperature (35 ± 2 °C for bacterial culture). Temperature in incubators should be recorded daily. Like all laboratory instruments, incubators must be cleaned regularly (at least every 14 days) and immediately after any infective material is spilt. Make sure that the actual temperature corresponds with the thermostat control when the instrument is used. In carbon dioxide incubators used for microbial culture, the concentration of carbon dioxide should be maintained at 5–10% and the humidity at 50–100%.

Water-baths

Water-baths are used for investigations at 25 °C, 30 °C, 37 °C, 42 °C, or 56 °C. It is important that the water-bath maintains a constant temperature within a narrow range (± 0.1 °C) during the investigation. Incorrect adjustment of the temperature and insufficient temperature stability will seriously affect the results of measurements.

Use of water-baths

1. The level of water in the water-bath must be above the level of the solution to be incubated.
2. Open containers, vials, or tubes must be incubated in a water-bath with the lid of the water-bath open to avoid contamination and dilution of the incubated material by condensed water.
3. The water in water-baths must be changed regularly to avoid the growth of algae and bacteria.

Periodic inspection and cleaning

- Circulators should be regularly disassembled and cleaned to remove scale and algae.
- Thermometers must be checked when they are received from the suppliers, and thereafter every 3 months, against a known standard (i.e., ice/water mixture or boiling water).
- The functioning of manometers must be checked every 3 months.

Balances

Balances are used to measure the weight or mass of a substance. If a comparison is made between two objects, one known and one unknown, then the measurement is mass. If the measurement is made against gravitational pull, then the measurement is weight.

There are two main categories of balance:

— mechanical balances,
— electromagnetic balances.

Balances that are based on other principles of measurement (e.g., piezoelectric balances, magneto-elastic balances, gyrodynamic balances, string balances) are less frequently used and will not be discussed here.

A number of factors influence the weighing processes. They become more important the smaller the mass of the substance to be measured. Therefore, the weighing of small quantities is more prone to errors than the weighing of large quantities.

The following influences can cause errors in measurement:

— temperature,
— moisture (atmospheric humidity),
— electrostatic effects,
— magnetism,
— gravitational forces,
— air,
— vibration.

Many analytical balances, and particularly those measuring in the microgram range, are constructed to minimize the effects of as many of these factors as possible.

The collective term "analytical balance" describes a balance suitable for chemical analysis. The weighing range of certified analytical balances is between 10 µg and 50 kg. They may be mechanical or electronic. Optical balances are mechanical balances equipped with an optical read-out.

Mechanical balances

Mechanical balances can be subdivided into:

- spring balances,
- sliding-weight balances,
- parallel-guidance-system balances,
- substitution balances:
    - three-knife substitution balances,
    - two-knife substitution balances.

With a spring balance the force of an object is compared with the known force of a spring. The calibration of a spring balance depends on the gravitational force on the object, which varies from one locality to another. Therefore spring balances must be calibrated at their place of use (Fig. 2.5).

Fig. 2.5. Spring balance.

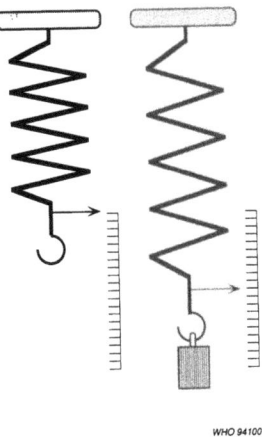

With a sliding-weight balance, the weight of an unknown object or substance is determined by a sliding device containing a known weight. Equilibrium is reached by displacement of the sliding weight along the runner, which is marked with scale divisions (household balance, Roman beam scale) (Fig. 2.6).

Fig. 2.6. Sliding-weight balance.

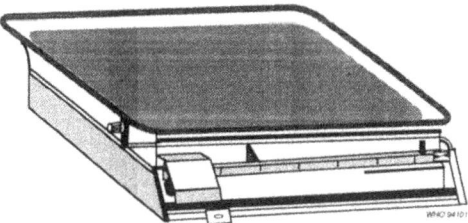

In a parallel-guidance-system balance, the degree of displacement of a beam from the equilibrium position is taken as a measure for an unknown mass. The parallel guidance prevents the weighing-pan from tipping over (letter balance) (Fig. 2.7).

In substitution balances, the sensitivity remains the same during measurement, since the beam always carries the same load on both sides, no matter what the load is. Substitution balances include equal-lever-arm balances (three-knife balances), and unequal-lever-arm balances (two-knife balances).

Fig. 2.7. Parallel-guidance balance.

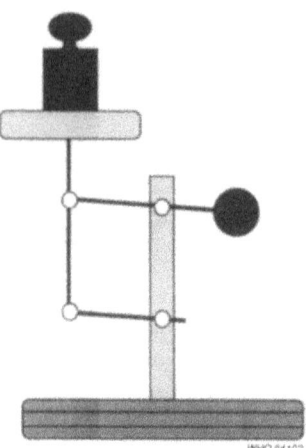

An equal-lever-arm balance has a symmetrical lever and three knife-edges—one in the centre and one at each end. The difference between two counter-rotating torques, generated by a known mass and an unknown mass, keeps the beam in a deflected position, which is taken as a measure for the unknown mass (Fig. 2.8).

Fig. 2.8. Equal-lever-arm balance.

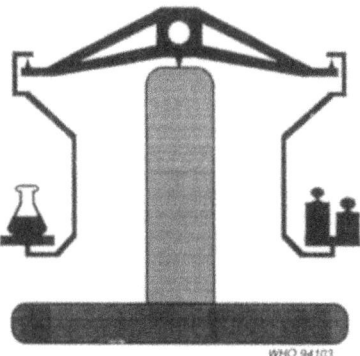

Unequal-lever-arm balances (two-knife balances) have one main knife-edge and a secondary knife-edge, which support both the load and the mass pieces, while a fixed counterweight is at the other end of the lever. If an unknown mass is placed on the pan, the balance beam deflects to that side. An appropriate number of masses must be removed from the side of the beam with the unknown load, so that the pointer returns to zero (Fig. 2.9).

Fig. 2.9. Unequal-lever-arm balance.

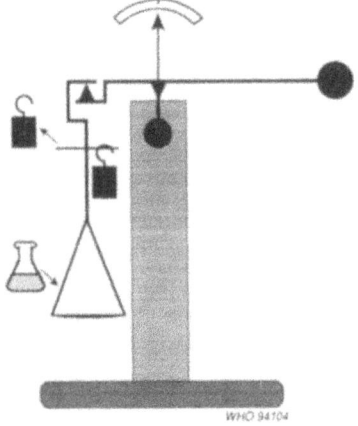

Electromagnetic balances

With an electromagnetic balance, the unknown mass is loaded on to a wire that is located between two poles of a permanent magnet, and to which an electrical circuit is applied (Fig. 2.10). The wire is mechanically displaced by the load. In order to bring the wire back to its original position, more current must be applied to the wire. The difference in the current required to keep the wire in the zero position when it is loaded and unloaded is proportional to, and taken as a measure of, the mass on the pan (Fig. 2.11).

Fig. 2.10. Electromagnetic balance, at rest.

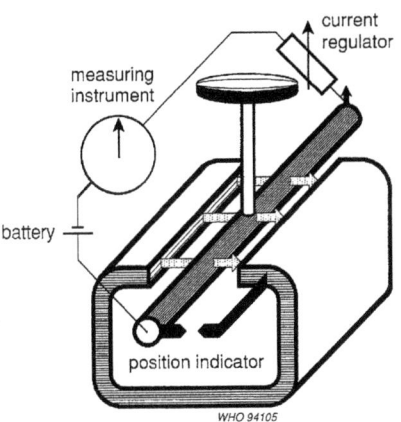

Fig. 2.11. Electromagnetic balance, under load.

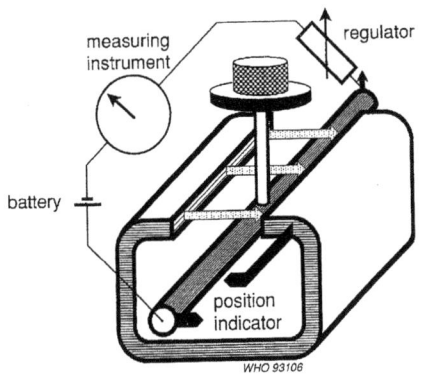

Good working practices—all balances

1. The balance must be zeroed prior to each use.
2. Always weigh chemicals/samples in a container, **never** directly on the pans.
3. Use the smallest possible container for weighing. Avoid containers made of plastic, because they can become electrostatically charged. Use glass vessels or weighing paper if possible. The weighing vessel and the sample to be weighed should be at the ambient temperature. Never put your hand into the weighing chamber, as this would cause the chamber to warm up.
4. Use clean weighing containers. Determine the mass of the weighing vessel prior to filling.
5. Place the sample in the weighing container, in the middle of the weighing pan to avoid corner-load error.
6. Keep the working-place, weighing chamber, and weighing-pan clean. Any spillage must be cleaned up immediately. Otherwise, chemicals may quickly corrode the balance, and biological materials may be a source of infection. Balance pans can be disinfected with 70% ethanol (700 ml/l).

Unpacking, siting, and installation

Read the manufacturer's instructions carefully.

1. With new or returned equipment, remove the packaging and any transit fixings that may have been fitted. Keep these safe for future use.
2. All balances should be sited on a solid, vibration-free surface that is free from draughts, away from sunlight, and at an even temperature. The atmosphere should be dust-free and chemical-free. **Never** store reagent bottles in a room with balances.
3. The instrument must be placed in a precisely horizontal position. This is checked using the spirit level. The air bubble must be in the centre of the level; if it is not centred, then a correction is made by turning the levelling-foot of the balance.
4. Before use or maintenance/repair, the balance must be levelled.

Hazards/safety

If good working practices are observed, there should be no special hazards. When simple balances have been used for weighing or balancing biological samples, it is prudent to disinfect the balance pans by swabbing with 70% ethanol (700 ml/l).

Special tools/spares/requirements

Leather cloth
Mini vacuum cleaner
Dust brush
Anti-magnetic tweezers
Watchmaker's screwdrivers
Dental mirror
Magnifying glass
Set of spanners to the manufacturer's specifications
Set of calibrating weights
Spare bulbs for optical balances.

Maintenance protocols

For all beam balances

1. Check balance is levelled.
2. Check that all control knobs are properly fitted.
3. Check zeroing device.
4. Check positioning of beam.
5. Check with both high and low mass calibrating weights.

For optical balances

As above for beam balances. Then:

- Make sure all counterbalancing weights are in place.
- Check with an appropriate milligram weight that the optical scale agrees with counterbalance weight.

For all balances

Service

- Tighten nuts and screws where applicable.
- Check and clean knife-edges.
- Check light path, clean, align, and focus.

Repair

- Read the manufacturer's service manual carefully, if it is available.
- With optical balances, remove covers and inspect beam and pivots for freedom of movement; gentle finger pressure on the pan may reveal a "sticky" linkage or bumper stop.

Check calibration

After any maintenance, service, repair, or re-siting.

Batteries

Batteries are energy sources that generate electrical energy from stored chemical energy. The electrical current results from the oxidation and reduction processes of the metals that are used as electrode materials in the battery cell. The tendency for oxidation (or reduction) differs from one metal to another. When two metal electrodes are immersed in a salt solution and are connected by an electrical conductor (wire), with a voltmeter in the circuit, the flow of electrons liberated at the surface of the metal electrodes can be measured as the potential difference (voltage). The quantity of electrical energy that can be made available is determined by the electrochemical potency of the metal electrodes and the concentration of the electrolyte solution. The reduction potentials of various metals are compared in Table 2.3.

Table 2.3. Standard reduction potentials of some metals at 25 °C

Metal	Reduction potential (V)
Silver (Ag/Ag$^+$)	− 0.22
Copper (Cu/Cu^{++})	− 0.34
Iron (Fe/Fe^{+++})	+ 0.0036
Lead (Pb/Pb^{++})	+ 0.13
Zinc (Zn/Zn^{++})	+ 0.76
Aluminium (Al/Al^{+++})	+ 1.66
Lead (Pb/Pb^{++})	− 1.46
Nickel (Ni/Ni^{++})	+ 0.23
Cadmium (Cd/Cd^{++})	+ 0.40
Lithium (Li/Li$^+$)	+ 3.05
Mercury (2Hg/Hg$_2^{++}$)	− 0.80

Batteries can be separated into primary and secondary systems. Primary systems can be used only once, because the active material required for the generation of electrical energy cannot be regenerated. Therefore, a primary system becomes useless once it has been discharged, and must be discarded.

Primary systems are mainly used in instruments for which the recharging of batteries is not practical. These systems are not suitable for instruments that have a relatively high requirement for electrical energy. Dry batteries are primary systems. The maximum voltage that can be produced by a dry battery is 1.5 volts per cell. The voltage decreases to 0.7 V during use. The electrical energy stored in alkaline dry batteries is about three times that stored in rechargeable nickel–cadmium batteries of the same size (see below). Dry batteries are used in instruments with a low and intermittent demand for electrical energy. Dry batteries should be stored separately when not being used. Most batteries of the primary type are either alkali–manganese batteries, or carbon–zinc batteries.

The most commonly used primary system battery is the carbon–zinc battery. It consists of a case made of zinc metal (Zn) as one electrode, a carbon rod coated with manganese oxide (MnO_2) as the other electrode, and an electrolyte solution of inspissated ammonium chloride (NH_4Cl). With this type of battery, the following chemical reactions generate the electricity:

Zinc electrode: $Zn \rightarrow Zn^{++} + 2e^-$

Carbon electrode: $2Mn^{IV}O_2 + 2H^+ + 2e^- \rightarrow 2Mn^{III}O(OH)$

The protons (H^+) are provided by the ammonium ions (NH_4^+).

In secondary systems, the chemical process for the generation of electrical energy is reversible, and the battery, once it has been discharged, can be recharged. Secondary systems can be used for instruments with greater requirements for electrical energy. The most common types are lead batteries and nickel–cadmium (Ni–Cd) batteries.

The term "battery" is conveniently used to describe a single, dry, electrochemical element or a coupled system of several electrochemical elements. In some languages the term "accumulator" is used for the coupled system. (For example, a car battery is often called a lead accumulator.)

Lead batteries

A lead battery is a liquid-system battery. The elements of a lead battery have narrow gratings filled with squamous lead (Pb) or squamous lead oxide (PbO_2) as electrodes. These electrodes are kept apart by a porous separator membrane. The electrolyte is 20–30% sulfuric acid. The following chemical reactions provide energy during electrical discharge:

Oxidation: $Pb + SO_4^{--} \rightarrow PbSO_4 + 2e^-$

Reduction: $PbO_2 + 4H^+ + SO_4^{--} + 2e^- \rightarrow PbSO_4 + 2H_2O$

These reactions go in the reverse direction when the battery is recharged.

Lead batteries are useful when a large capacity is required and a continuous supply of electricity is not reliably available. A 12 volt car battery or two 6 volt batteries can be used to supply any of the instruments in a hospital that run on 12 volts direct current. Many instruments can run on lead batteries, for example room illumination, water pumps, refrigerators, and mechanical tools. Lead batteries can be recharged from the mains supply, or by a photovoltaic solar-powered system independently of the mains.

Use of lead batteries

A lead battery must be protected from overcharge, because of water loss from the cells. It must also be protected from too heavy a discharge since this will drastically shorten the life of the battery. The battery can be checked by measuring the voltage with a multimeter. This check also gives information about the actual capacity of the battery.

For a 12 volt lead battery to be recharged at an ambient temperature of 30 °C the limit values are:

– maximum voltage for recharge: 13.9 volt (additional charging will cause high losses of water)
– minimum voltage for recharge: 11.2 volt.

The battery should be recharged when it has a residual capacity of about 30%. Additional discharge shortens the life of the battery considerably.

Table 2.4 shows the energy that can be supplied from a 12 V, 100 ampere-hour (Ah), lead battery in relation to the discharge current.

Table 2.4. Relation between maximum capacity of a lead battery and discharge current

Time for discharge (hours)	Discharge current (amperes)	Maximum capacity (ampere-hours)
100	1.0	100
50	1.8	90
20	4.2	84
10	8.0	80
5	14.0	70
2	25.0	50

Typically, the difference in voltage between a completely charged (100%) and a 50% charged lead battery is only 0.3 V. The capacity is determined by measuring the density of the sulfuric acid in the cells. Table 2.5 shows the densities that are valid for tropical countries.

Table 2.5. Densities of sulfuric acid and respective battery capacity (for tropical countries)

Density of H_2SO_4 (kg/litre)	Battery capacity (%)
1.23	100
1.16	50
1.10	0

Exhausted lead batteries can be identified by measuring their voltage under working conditions, that is before and after use. The higher the difference in voltage, the less the battery can be loaded.

When new lead batteries are filled with distilled water and sulfuric acid, it is important that the acid is added to the water slowly. The water should never be added to the acid, as this will cause heating and may lead to sudden splashing of the mixture. The density of the diluted sulfuric acid should be 1.23 kg/litre in tropical countries.

Recharging lead–acid batteries

1. Standard lead–acid batteries must be checked every month to ensure that the electrolyte solution in each battery is at the correct level. When the level is low, distilled water must be added. If distilled water is not available, consult the manufacturer. Some kinds of bottled water are satisfactory, and freshly collected rainwater, free from sediment or foreign particles, can be used in an emergency. The amount of water added to each battery, or each section of the battery, should be recorded, with the date. If one battery requires more than the others, the maintenance service should be informed at once.
2. Sealed lead–acid batteries need checking every month. All have an indicator on top, often a blue or red spot that changes if the battery is failing. At the first indication of failure, inform the maintenance service at once. Do not wait for the battery to fail completely.
3. Batteries should be recharged as soon as they are discharged; they must not be left discharged for long periods.
4. It is good practice to limit the recharging current to approximately 7 A for a battery rated at 100 A h, and 3.5 A for a battery rated at 50 A h.
5. Do not allow the electrolyte temperature to rise above 38 °C if the normal room temperature is below 32 °C, or above 40 °C if the normal room temperature is above 32 °C. If the temperature does rise above this limit, stop charging and let the battery cool down.
6. Carry on charging until all the cells are bubbling freely, and the specific gravities and cell voltages have stopped rising, measured by 3 readings over 3 hours.
7. Do not top-up the battery with tapwater unless there is really no alternative. Use distilled water instead. You should be able to make your own by cooling steam and collecting the condensate.
8. Keep the outside of the battery clean. Damp and grease on the top surface can cause electrical discharge (tracking) between the terminals.
9. Do not allow a battery to remain in a very cold place for long. If it must be used in an unheated area, try to insulate it, but at the same time allow free movement of air around the top to allow the gas produced to disperse.
10. Do not use a battery charger that recharges very quickly, except as a last resort. This can damage the plates.
11. Check the level of the sulfuric acid at least every 6 months. Refill the battery with distilled water if necessary.
12. The battery-pack used as a generator in X-ray equipment stores a very powerful electric charge, sufficient to cause severe injuries, or even death in some cases.

    – Never touch the battery-pack—even the outside of the box—with wet hands or when there is any liquid on the floor or nearby.
    – If you have to open the battery-pack, remove any metallic jewellery, including watches and rings. Do not wear a necklace that may hang down as you bend over. Do not have any metallic object (money, a pen, a knife, or a metal comb) in your pocket that might fall out into the pack.
    – If you use tools, all must be fully insulated.
    – Do not touch any wires inside the pack unless they are fully insulated, your hands are dry, and there is no water or liquid on the floor,

Nickel–cadmium (Ni–Cd) batteries

Ni–Cd batteries are storage batteries, like lead–acid batteries, and work on a different electrochemical principle from alkaline and carbon–zinc batteries, over which they have some advantages.

- Ni–Cd batteries are lighter than carbon–zinc batteries, while being more powerful.
- Ni–Cd batteries can be repeatedly recharged and require little maintenance.

Ni–Cd batteries have the following components:

- a negative electrode (cadmium),
- a positive electrode (nickel), and
- electrolyte (KOH).

In addition, the battery contains a separator that binds the electrolyte, and isolates the electrodes. The quality of a Ni–Cd battery is determined primarily by the quality of the electrodes.

Ni–Cd batteries are constructed as open systems or closed gas-tight units. A single Ni–Cd cell has a potential difference of 1.25 volts. The actual voltage fluctuates between 1.4 and 1.2 volts when the battery is in use. On complete discharge, the voltage drops to 1.0 volt. Several cells must be connected in series if a high voltage is required. Sometimes cells are connected in parallel to achieve a higher discharge capacity. For this purpose special care must be taken that they are gas-tight. Ni–Cd systems cannot be recharged when coupled in parallel.

The technical characteristics of the most common Ni-Cd batteries are shown in Table 2.6.

Table 2.6. Technical characteristics of Ni–Cd batteries

Type	Capacity (mAh)	Recharge current (mA)	Maximum continuous load (A)	Pulse load for 2 seconds (A)
Mono D	4000	400	28	90
Baby C	1800	180	18	72
Mignon AA	500	50	3	10
Micro AAA	180	18	1	3.6
Lady N	150	15	0.6	2

Gas-tight Ni–Cd batteries

High pressures can develop inside a gas-tight battery following inappropriate handling or use. Such high internal pressures can damage the battery, and can result in hazards for personnel. Therefore most gas-tight Ni–Cd batteries are constructed with a pressure valve that opens automatically to release any excess of gas that develops during the electrochemical reaction. The pressure valve opens at a pressure of between 900 and 1800 kPa. Some valves shut again automatically when the internal pressure is reduced.

Use of Ni–Cd batteries at elevated ambient temperatures

Problems may arise when Ni–Cd batteries are used in hot climates. They are sometimes unreliable because of an increased rate of discharge, and less efficient recharging at higher ambient temperatures. These problems may be partially overcome by following the simple rules outlined below.

Recharging

Ni–Cd batteries should be recharged:

– shortly before use
– at low ambient temperatures (e.g., in a refrigerator or a specially constructed case, if necessary).

The performance of a fully charged Ni–Cd battery charged at different ambient temperatures is indicated in Table 2.7.

Table 2.7. Percentage of energy available from Ni–Cd batteries charged at different temperatures

Ambient temperature (°C)	Percentage of energy available
20	87
30	77
40	62
50	35

Example: 62% of the energy can be made available from a Ni–Cd battery that was charged at 40 °C.

Storage

Ni–Cd batteries must be stored at a low temperature in an insulated, dry container.

The residual capacity (% available energy) of a Ni–Cd battery stored at different temperatures is indicated in Table 2.8.

Table 2.8. Residual capacity of Ni–Cd batteries stored at different temperatures

Duration of storage	Temperature (°C)			
	20	30	40	60
1 week	83	77	60	45
2 weeks	72	60	32	7
3 weeks	60	38		

Example: A Ni–Cd battery stored under dry conditions for 2 weeks at 40 °C would have a residual capacity of 32%. High humidity accelerates the discharge of the battery.

Ni–Cd batteries can be recharged in 14 hours using mains electricity and an appropriate recharger. If the electric power system is not reliable, a photovoltaic recharge system can be used; smaller batteries can be recharged in this way within 1 sunny day. More recently, special rechargers have been developed that require 11–32 volts for recharging. They can be used to connect a Ni–Cd battery to a car battery for recharging.[1]

---

[1] Obtainable from Solenco GmbH, POB 100 219, 4019 Monheim, Germany.

Control of capacity

The technique for measuring the capacity of a Ni–Cd battery is complicated. However, the following methods have been found to be practical.

- Voltage measurement with a multimeter. However, the results are difficult to interpret because the difference between complete charge and total discharge is only 0.24 V.
- Use of a battery test system.
- Voltage measurement prior to and after a load of 10 times the stated recharging current of the battery. A fully charged new battery will show only a minor difference, while an old battery will give a reading of not more than 1.0 volt after the load.

Notes on batteries

Before buying, or accepting as a gift, a piece of equipment that uses batteries, check that replacements are readily available. Also, remember that batteries are expensive to buy and can be difficult to store satisfactorily. Sometimes, mains or low-voltage powered equipment might be a better option.

When the equipment is not in use remove the batteries, to avoid possible corrosion and damage to the instrument.

Cell counters

Cell counters are used for haematological measurement. Semi-automated and automated cell counting has proved to be much more reliable than microscopic cell counting, because a far greater number of cells can be counted rapidly in a specimen by an analyser system, resulting in greater precision. However, the improvement in precision does not necessarily imply a simultaneous improvement in accuracy. For the study of pathological cell types, microscopic examination of a blood smear by an experienced investigator is still most valuable, and in many instances the method of choice.

A number of different principles are used in cell analysers:

– impedance measurement,
– light scattering,
– centrifugation and quantitative buffy-coat analysis.

Using these techniques, all major classes of blood cells (erythrocytes, platelets, leukocytes) can be identified and even subclasses (granulocytes and lymphocytes) can be measured. More sophisticated instruments, which combine measurement of cell size and cell fluorescence, or cell size determination and immunofluorescence, allow subclassification.

Impedance measurement is most commonly used for cell counting. This principle of measurement takes advantage of the fact that blood cells are less conductive than the diluent electrolyte. The principle of the method is explained below.

1. When an electrical potential is applied to two electrodes dipped into an electrolyte solution, an electric current can be measured owing to the transport of ions from one electrode to the other. The magnitude of the current will depend on the concentration of the ions in solution. It will be constant if the transport of ions is constant (Fig. 2.12a).
2. If the electrodes are separated by an insulator, the flow of electric current will drop to zero (Fig. 2.12b).

Fig. 2.12. Measurement of impedance as a method of counting cells.

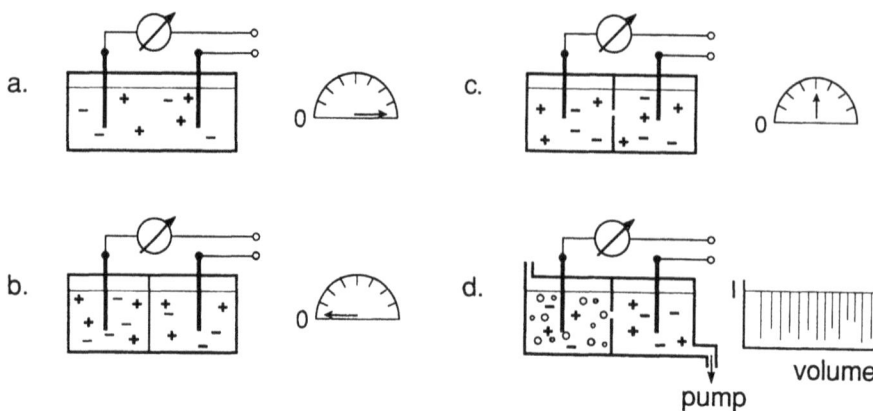

3. The current will reappear if a small aperture is introduced into the insulator, but the magnitude of the current will be small, because the insulation is still partially effective (Fig. 2.12c).
4. A small particle such as a blood cell with a conductivity lower than that of the electrolyte solution, passing through the aperture from one chamber to another, will temporarily decrease the current because a smaller volume of the electrolyte solution is able to pass through the aperture at the same time. The current will regain its original value when the particle has passed through the aperture (Fig. 2.12d).

When a cell-containing fluid is sucked through the aperture of an insulator separating two electrode chambers, each change in current (registered as a pulse) indicates the passage of a particle through the aperture, thus allowing the cells to be counted. Furthermore, the magnitude of each pulse is proportional to the size of the particle. Simple cell counters register only the number of pulses above a certain threshold. More sophisticated counters also register the magnitude of each pulse and show the distribution of the pulse magnitudes, thus indicating the distribution of particle sizes in the population of cells. The concentration of cells in the sample is measured by counting the number of pulses for a known volume of fluid.

The principle of measurement implies that each measured pulse is attributed to the passage of a single particle through the aperture of the separating membrane. Therefore, a blood specimen having a cell concentration of about 5 million cells per microlitre must be appropriately diluted (in general, 200- or 250-fold) to ensure that individual cells are counted. Sometimes, errors resulting from the passage of more than one cell still occur in specimens with high cell concentrations. These errors can be avoided by:

– Further dilution of the blood specimen and a repeat measurement.
– Application of a correction factor to the number of cells counted to allow for coincidence. This factor varies with the cell concentration and may be taken from a table provided for the instrument by the manufacturer. Modern instruments have a built-in calculation programme to allow for coincidence.

Most cell counters cannot be calibrated by the user. Therefore, a standard prepared, or purchased, cell suspension can serve only for control of precision but not for accuracy. The given cell concentration in commercially available control materials can be used only for measurement with a specified instrument; different results will be obtained with instruments with a different threshold limit.

The determination of cell size by impedance measurement is influenced by a number of technical factors, which may vary from one instrument to another, and also by the type and shape of the particles being measured. For example, the magnitude of the signal from a discoid cell, e.g., an erythrocyte, is different from that from a spherical cell, e.g., a leukocyte, even if the cells have the same volume.

Cell counters using the impedance principle count the combined total of red blood cells which have a cell volume between 70 and 120 fl (femtolitres), and leukocytes, which have a cell volume between 100 and 350 fl. The results are given in terms of red blood cell count, ignoring the negligible proportion of leukocytes (usually only 0.2%—10 000 leukocytes compared with 5 million red cells per ml). However, a considerable error may occur in specimens with a much higher proportion of leukocytes, e.g. those from patients with pronounced anaemia and high leukocyte concentrations.

For leukocyte counting, erythrocytes are lysed by an ionic or non-ionic detergent in solution—a procedure that does not lyse leukocytes within a certain time. However, the size of the leukocytes, and particularly of the polymorphonuclear cells, may vary. Erroneously low counts may be obtained at high leukocyte concentrations, when for example two cells pass through the aperture simultaneously, while being registered only as a single pulse. Such errors can be eliminated by greater dilution of the specimen, as mentioned above.

Measurement of platelet concentration is more prone to error, because of their small cell size (1–10 fl). It is particularly important that the buffer solution used for the dilution of the blood specimen is free of dust particles; these solutions must be filtered through a filter of 1 μm pore size. Absence of dust is also important for counting of red and white blood cells, although the presence of impurities with a particle size of less than 1 μm is of less importance.

General errors that will affect measurements of cell concentrations are:

- unsatisfactory blood sampling and storage;
- inadequate dilution of the specimen;
- fibrin precipitates or cryoprecipitates in the specimen;
- inadequate lysis of red blood cells when counting white blood cells;
- lack of homogeneity in the distribution of blood cells in the dilution.

Technical errors in cell counting may result from:

- fluctuations in the electric current;
- incorrect setting of the size threshold of the instrument;
- dust particles in the diluent;
- leakage in the suction system of the instrument;
- partial or total obstruction of the aperture;
- multiple cell passage at high cell counts;
- carry-over from one measurement to a subsequent measurement.

To avoid these errors, the following measures must be routinely undertaken:

- the cell counter should be connected to an electrical stabilizer;
- the aperture between the electrolyte chambers should be checked after each series of measurements, and cleaned with a small soft brush, if necessary;
- the electrodes must be checked, to ensure that they dip into the electrolyte solution in both chambers;
- the fittings of removable parts should be coated with silicone grease to avoid air-leakage in the suction system;
- the bottle of diluent solution should be checked daily, and the waste solution discarded;
- the suction system should be cleaned with diluent solution to avoid carry-over effects;

– at the end of each working day, the suction system should be cleaned with detergent solution and afterwards with the diluent solution;
– the aperture of the glass cuvette must always be kept immersed in diluent solution to avoid obstruction.

Further maintenance procedures (e.g., cleaning of mercury, etc.), must be carried out according to the manufacturer's instructions.

Centrifuges

Basic principles

A centrifuge is a machine that applies a sustained centrifugal force (i.e., a force due to rotation) to impel matter outwards from the centre of rotation. This principle is used to separate out particles in a liquid medium by sedimentation. The physical basis of the separation is the action of a centrifugal force on the rotating particles, which increases with the radius of the rotational field and the velocity of the rotation. The rate of sedimentation is determined by the density of the particles. Dense particles sediment first, followed by lighter particles. Depending on the conditions, very light particles may even remain in suspension.

The relative centrifugal force is related to the number of revolutions of the rotor per minute according to the formula:

$$\text{RCF} = 1.118 \times 10^{-6} \times r \times n^2$$

where RCF = relative centrifugal force (g)

r = radius in millimetres from the centrifuge spindle to point of tube, and

n = no. of revolutions per minute.

The relative centrifugal force can easily be calculated from a nomogram (Fig. 2.13), where the radius is measured from the centre of the rotor to the middle of the tube placed in the radially oriented rotor bucket; e.g., if the radius is 75 mm, the speed of rotation must be 2500 revolutions per minute to develop a centrifugal force of 520 g. It is important that the temperature in the centrifuge does not exceed 37 °C, otherwise degradation of some constituents of the specimen may occur.

There are two main types of centrifuge: preparative and analytical.

Preparative centrifuges are used to separate the solids suspended in biological samples from the supporting fluid. This is the most common type of centrifuge, and they are fitted with swing-out, or fixed-angle, heads.

Preparative centrifuges vary in their sample capacity and size, from floor-standing to small capacity centrifuges that can be sited on a bench. Some are fitted with internal wind shields to protect the operator from contamination by any aerosols that may be formed. This is now a mandatory safety requirement in many countries.

Two types of preparative centrifuge are currently used—mechanical and electrical—although the majority are electrical centrifuges.

Analytical centrifuges may be used to quantify one or more solid components in a mixed suspension. The only centrifuge of this type used in medical laboratories is the microhaematocrit centrifuge.

Fig. 2.13. Nomogram for determination of the relative centrifugal force.

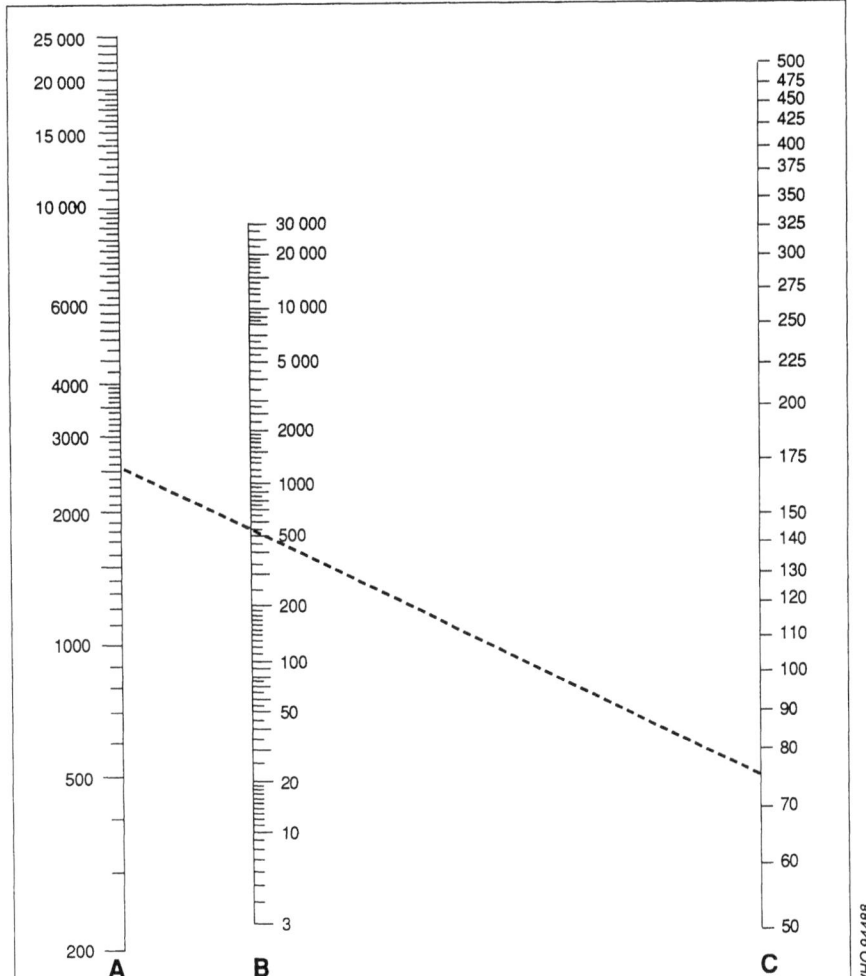

A Speed of centrifuge spindle in rpm.
B Relative centrifugal force (x g).
C Radius in mm from centre of centrifuge spindle to point along tube or flask.

Unpacking, siting, installation, and electrical requirements

Follow the manufacturer's instructions, if these are available. Remove all packing and any transit fixings that may have been used.

Check that the equipment voltage is the same as the local supply, and that the fuse rating is correct. A correct fuse should protect the equipment from serious electrical damage.

Both bench and floor-standing centrifuges must be sited on a rigid surface, away from laboratory balances. Bench centrifuges should be at least 20 cm from the edge of the bench. If the sample breaks during rotation, considerable "out of balance" forces are generated, and the centrifuge may move about unpredictably.

Good working practices

Preparative centrifuges

- The centrifuge must be positioned exactly horizontally to avoid movement if the instrument is out of balance during operation.
- It is critically important that the centrifuge load is balanced at all times. Therefore, tubes should be loaded in matched buckets fitted with rubber cushions, and should be arranged so that like loads are opposite. A "dummy", i.e., a tube containing the appropriate volume of water, must be included when an odd number of specimens are to be centrifuged. Final balancing should be carried out by placing paired loads on the two pans of a reasonably sensitive balance, and balancing by adding water from a bottle or Pasteur pipette; if possible, add water to the lighter of the two samples, so that it balances the heavier load. Biological samples should be capped during centrifugation. The centrifuge should be stopped immediately if it develops an abnormal noise, indicating that it is not properly balanced.
- After use the buckets should be inverted to drain dry.
- After any sample spillage, always clean up the buckets and the centrifuge and disinfect with 70% (700 ml/l) alcohol immediately.
- Clean and disinfect the centrifuge often, because it is one of the most frequently used instruments.
- Check mountings and replace if necessary.
- Check motor brushes and replace if necessary.
- Check for corrosion and clean if necessary.
- Never operate a centrifuge with the lid open.
- Do not use the centrifuge at higher speeds than necessary.

Haematocrit centrifuges

Haematocrit centrifuges need not be balanced before use. As the samples are small capillary tubes, and the forces relatively low, it is only necessary to load the samples symmetrically. Never run the centrifuge with the lid open. Capillaries should be plugged at one end with the recommended sealing compound. The plugged end should always be placed against the sealing gasket. Even with the above precautions, it is possible that blood may leak from the bottom of the capillary. After any spillage, the centrifuge chamber must be disinfected and cleaned immediately with soap solution, and then with 70% (700 ml/l) alcohol.

Hazards/safety

Because centrifuges are regularly used to prepare blood and urine samples, it is recommended that the rotor bowl, centrifuge head, buckets and trunnion rings be disinfected before any servicing is carried out.

Tools

A general tool kit is satisfactory.

Spares

Suppression capacitor (interference filter)
Carbon brushes
Rubber feet (bench models)

Rubber cushions (for preparative centrifuges)
Sealing gasket (for haematocrit centrifuges)

Maintenance

1. Check lid lock.
2. Inspect trunnion rings and buckets for metal fatigue.
3. Check hinges, control knobs, rubber feet.
4. Check the weight of the buckets and replace them in their holders. The rubber cushions in the buckets may be lost or taken out for cleaning and misplaced, so that uneven loads occur. Even small weight differences can cause rapid wear and degradation of the motor bearings.

Service

1. Inspect brakes for proper operation.
2. Adjust lid lock to ensure proper operation of the electrical interlock.
3. Check for loose connections.
4. Check carbon brushes for wear, or lack of spring tension.
5. Check timer (if fitted).
6. Grease motor bearings.

Calibration

This is not generally required on preparative centrifuges. Haematocrit centrifuges may be checked with a tachometer, if one is available.

Electrode equipment

Electrodes are used for measuring the electrical potential that develops when a strip of metal is immersed in a dilute solution of a gas or salts. A transfer of gases or ions between the metal and the solution occurs, establishing the electrical potential (see also "Batteries" p. 13). The magnitude of the potential varies with the concentration of ions in the solution. If two electrodes are dipped into a solution, the difference between the electrical potentials of the two electrodes can be measured (Fig. 2.14). If one of the electrodes has a stable potential (i.e., a reference electrode), measurement of the potential difference can be used to determine the gas or ion concentration in the solution.

Fig. 2.14. Potentiometric chain.

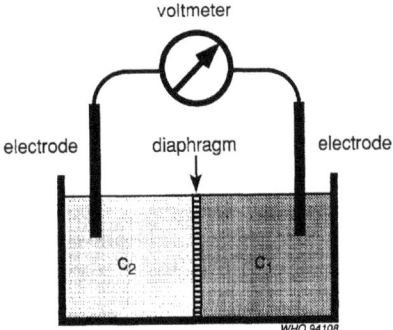

The physical basis of electrical potential is described by a linear equation, as first shown by Nernst:

$$E = E_o + \frac{RT}{n.F} \times \ln a$$

where:

- E = measured voltage,
- E_o = baseline potential (of a 1 mol/litre solution at room temperature),
- R = gas constant (8.3144 J/(K·mol)),
- T = temperature (Kelvin),
- n = charge number of the ion to be measured,
- F = Faraday constant (96 485 coulombs/mol),
- a = activity of the ion or gas to be measured (in dilute solutions a is close to the gas or ion concentration).

Electrode characteristics

The characteristics of an electrode can be described by a diagram showing the electrode voltage that is measured when it is immersed with a reference electrode in salt solutions of known concentrations. When the electrical potential is plotted against the logarithm of concentration, the resulting curve has a linear section (Fig. 2.15), the slope of which can be calculated by the following equation:

$$S = (E_1 - E_2)/(\log c_1 - \log c_2)$$
$$= (E_1 - E_2)/\log c_1/c_2$$

where S = slope,
E_1 = electrode potential in salt solution 1,
E_2 = electrode potential in salt solution 2,
c_1 = ion concentration in salt solution 1,
c_2 = ion concentration in salt solution 2.

Fig. 2.15. Relation between voltage and ion concentration in electrode measurement.

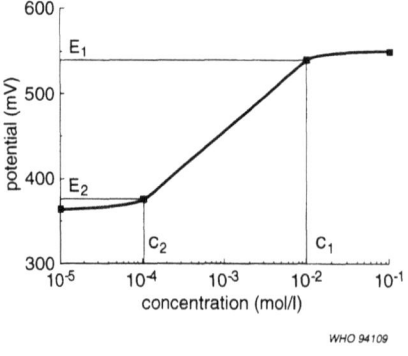

The slope is a measure of the sensitivity of an electrode and has the dimension of voltage. The slopes of the curves obtained with different electrodes will vary according to their ionic sensitivity.

In a system in which the ion concentration in salt solution 1 is 10 times higher than that in salt solution 2, $\log (c_1/c_2) = \log 10 = 1$, and the equation for calculating the slope becomes:

$$S = E_1 - E_2.$$

The slope of the electrode potential curve will change with the temperature of measurement and with the charge number of the ion to be measured. The temperature dependence of the slope for an electrode with a high sensitivity, used for measurement of an ideal monovalent ion, will be near the values shown below:

Temperature (°C)	Slope (mV)
0	54.19
10	56.18
20	58.16
25	59.15
30	60.14
40	62.13

By using ion-selective membranes or other devices, it is possible to design electrodes that are specific for the measurement of one analyte in a solution containing a mixture of analytes. In laboratory medicine, this method has been used to measure H^+ (pH), Na^+, K^+, Li^+, Ca^{++}, CO_2, O_2, glucose, urea, and a number of other analytes. However, for many of these analytes, the use of selective electrodes is expensive and the equipment is difficult to maintain at a level that gives satisfactory analytical precision. It is therefore recommended that electrodes should be used mainly for the measurement of pH and blood gas analysis (CO_2, O_2). Equipment is commercially available for the measurement of Na^+ and K^+ using ion-selective electrodes, but this technique is not superior to flame photometry, which is still the method of reference (see p. 29).

pH meters

The concentration of hydrogen ions in a solution, which is conveniently expressed in terms of its negative decadic logarithm, pH, is often measured during the preparation of reagent solutions or buffer systems, and also in clinical blood gas analysis.

For the measurement of hydrogen ion concentration, a glass electrode is used in most pH meters. Glass electrodes are made from special types of glass that allow hydrogen ions to be absorbed and to penetrate into deeper layers of the glass. Other small ions, such as lithium and sodium ions, may also be absorbed to some extent and change the properties of the electrode, causing the so-called "salt error". Glass electrodes are suitable for measurement in the range pH 0–11. In solutions with a pH above 11, the salt error becomes important and results in readings of pH that are too low. In an ideal electrode, the potential difference is 59.1 mV/pH unit at 25 °C. This value is used to calibrate a pH meter in terms of pH units. Since potential difference depends on temperature, pH measurements should be made at the calibration temperature; otherwise a correction factor must be applied.

Calomel (dimercury chloride) electrodes are used as reference electrodes. They establish a constant potential in an aqueous solution which is independent of the pH in the solution. Their potential alters only at very low pH (pH < 1), and then only slightly.

For the calibration of a pH meter, special buffer solutions must be used; the pH of the buffer should be near the pH of the solution to be measured. Phosphate buffers and acetate buffers are preferable. Problems may occur with alkaline buffers, since their pH may decrease with the absorption of CO_2 from the air. This is why all calibration buffers must be sealed during storage.

Installation

Blood-gas analysers and pH meters should be located in a clean environment, away from any area where dangerous or corrosive chemicals are stored. For the calibration of blood-gas analysers, supplies of oxygen and carbon dioxide are required, and they should therefore be sited appropriately.

Electrodes should be used as recommended for the specified purpose, and the recommended procedure for equilibration should be followed when new electrodes are installed. New glass electrodes must be soaked in a buffer solution (pH 4–8) for at least 24 hours before use to obtain a stable potential. They should be calibrated at two values, using the manufacturer's calibration materials or solutions prepared from pH buffer tablets. If these are not readily available, buffer solutions should be prepared for the purpose. However, these solutions should be checked from time to time against the manufacturer's calibrants or solutions prepared from pH buffer tablets.

Manufacturer's calibration solutions should be used to calibrate blood-gas analysers and the usual clinical/chemical quality control procedures should be used to monitor day-to-day performance.

Good practice

- Keep instrument clean.
- Cover after use.
- Rinse electrode after use. For short-term storage, it may be kept in a plastic beaker filled with distilled water to prevent damage.
- Check contact between electrode, plug, and instrument.
- Avoid contact between electrode and glass beaker.
- If applicable, remove the rubber stopper during measurement and refit to electrode after use.
- Make sure that the electrode is always filled with electrolyte according to the manufacturer's instructions.
- Do not touch the electrode membrane, since it can be easily damaged.
- Glass electrodes should be kept immersed in a standard salt solution for long-term storage. Reference electrodes should be kept in a standard salt solution during storage for short intervals, and should be stored dry, with a protective cap, for long-term storage. Glass electrodes that have been stored dry must be soaked in 0.1 mol/litre HCl for at least 4 hours. Thereafter, they must be carefully washed with distilled water.
- Calomel electrodes must be kept in a potassium chloride (KCl) buffer solution after use. They must always contain some KCl crystals.
- Protein precipitates on the electrode must be carefully removed by digestion with pepsin solutions, at pH 2 for a few hours. Thereafter, the electrode must be rinsed thoroughly with distilled water.

Glass electrodes will usually maintain their properties for many years if used appropriately and stored correctly. Aging of an electrode is indicated when a constant potential does not develop within a few seconds after insertion into an ionic solution.

A calomel electrode should be considered unsatisfactory if two calomel electrodes, when filled with the same KCl solution, differ by more than 5 mV when measured in the same pH meter.

In modern blood-gas analysers, in which the electrodes are an integral part of the instrument, some of these precautions will not be applicable.

Repairs

If electrodes are stored incorrectly the membrane may dry out. It is sometimes possible to restore performance by removing the outer layer of the membrane with a smooth flat file.

Hazards

If electrodes are used for measuring biological fluids, they must be cleaned and disinfected according to the manufacturer's recommendations.

Packing

Electrodes are very fragile and must therefore be packed correctly, following the manufacturer's instructions. Care is needed in removing the packaging.

Flame photometers

Flame photometers are used routinely for the measurement of lithium (Li), sodium (Na), and potassium (K) in body fluids. More sophisticated instruments can also measure calcium (Ca).

In flame photometry, an aqueous salt solution is dispersed in air. The salt in the dispersed droplets is transferred into a gaseous state by heating with a flame, and then quickly disintegrates into gaseous atoms. Above a critical temperature the atoms absorb energy, which excites the electrons into higher energy states. When the excited electrons return to their original state, they emit the absorbed energy as light. The wavelength of the light emitted by each metal is characteristic for that element. The intensity of the light emitted at the given wavelength is proportional to the number of excited metal atoms and can be measured with a suitable optical filter and photodetector.

This principle—also called flame emission photometry—can be used to measure more than 50 elements. However, it is mainly used for determination of the alkali metals, the excitation of which requires only a low energy input from a low-temperature flame (propane/air or butane/air).

Under ideal circumstances, there is a linear correlation between the concentration of the element in dispersion and the light intensity at a specific wavelength. However, in practice, there will be some degree of ionization, depending on the concentration of the element. Additionally, the presence of other elements may suppress ionization. Both atoms and ions of an element in the gaseous state can be excited, but the emission spectra from atoms and ions are different. Therefore, it is necessary to choose conditions of measurement in which only atom emission spectra are obtained. The optimal conditions must be defined for each element. When measuring potassium in a specimen, for example, the addition of another element, such as lithium, to the solution not only suppresses potassium ionization, but can at the same time provide internal calibration, if the lithium concentration is measured with a reference detector. A flame photometer with a reference detector for lithium therefore compensates for fluctuations in the energy input from the flame.

A flame photometer consists of the following essential parts (Fig. 2.16):

– nebulizer
– burner

- filter and optics
- detector and multiplier
- air compressor
- gas supply.

Fig. 2.16. Flame photometer assembly.

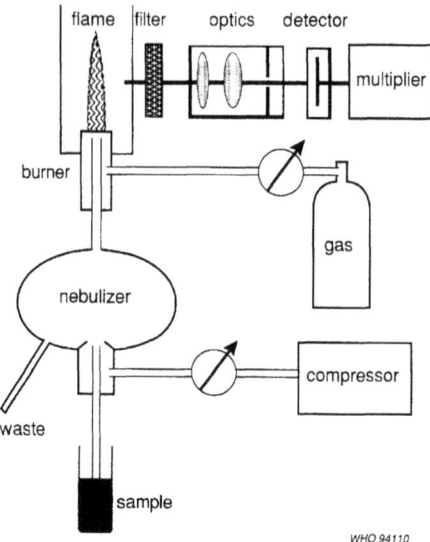

The specimen solution is mixed with a diluent which may contain a lithium salt at a defined concentration. Many flame photometers have a dilutor as an integral part of the instrument. This diluted solution is dispersed by compressed air in the nebulizer chamber, and heated in a gas flame. The emitted light passes through the optical system to the detector.

The filter wavelengths for measurement are:

Li—671 nm
Na—589 nm
K—768 nm

With a well maintained flame photometer, the coefficient of variation in measurement can be as low as 1.5% for Li and 0.5% for Na and K.

Services required

In addition to a reliable electricity supply, flame photometers require:

- compressed air at a pressure of about 100 kPa, from either an electrically powered air compressor or a gas cylinder (but this is expensive);
- a gas cylinder connected to the flame photometer through an air filter, or a gas supply (city gas, butane, or propane), as specified by the manufacturer;
- distilled water;
- drainage point.

Unpacking, siting, installation

1. Read the manufacturer's instructions carefully.
2. Remove the instrument from its packing and wipe the external surfaces with a cloth. Keep the packing for possible future use.

3. Install the instrument on a vibration-free bench, away from direct sunlight and draughts.
4. Place the air compressor on the floor, or on a purpose-built shelf, as compressors cause much vibration (and noise).
5. Ensure that the operating voltage of the flame photometer and compressor is the same as the local supply.
6. Following the manufacturer's instructions, connect the gas supply, the compressed air supply, and the drainage tube to the flame photometer.
7. If the instrument has removable optical filters, put these in place. **Never** use the flame photometer without the filters in place.
8. Some instruments with meters have a locking device. Unlock this before use.

Operation and maintenance

Since the degree of dilution of the specimen and the gas pressure are critical, it is advisable to follow the operating instructions for the instrument supplied by the manufacturer.

For most instruments, measurements can be made on serum. However, serum protein may precipitate in the tubes and dilution chamber. Similarly, the burner, the burning chamber (chimney), and the filter can become contaminated by such particles if the gas and air mixture does not provide complete combustion.

The following precautions should be noted:

- Samples should be homogeneous, and not highly viscous.
- Check the performance of the instrument with a calibrator and a quality control serum prior to each series of measurements on unknown specimens. Calibrators and samples must be diluted with the same diluent.
- Check the gas bottles daily.
- Adjust the air supply from the compressor as recommended by the manufacturer.
- Clean the tubing and nebulizer system by suction of distilled water after each series of measurements. Leakage in the system can be checked by use of a soap solution; this may also clean precipitates from tubing. Dilutors with a pumping system, using rubber tubing, must be checked routinely at frequent intervals, since the tubing will soften after prolonged use, leading to problems in measurement due to erratic dilution of the specimen.
- Turn off the gas supply after each run.
- Empty the waste container daily.
- Clean the tubing of the dilutor and nebulizer weekly, and rinse with distilled water.
- Clean the burner, glass chimney, and filters every 6 months with a lint-free cloth, a cleaning solution, and methanol.

Remember: Optical filters must be handled only by the edges.

Good working practices

Follow the manufacturer's operating instructions:

- Check that the gas cylinder is sufficiently full.
- Check that the working pressure of the gas cylinder is correct.
- Never operate the photometer without the optical filters in place.

Clean the flame photometer by aspirating distilled water through the atomizer after each series of measurements.

When switching off:

1. Turn off the gas.
2. Wait for extinction of the flame.
3. Turn off the air.
4. Remove the distilled water from the aspiration line.
5. Switch off the instrument and the compressor.
6. Allow to cool.
7. Cover with plastic cover to keep out dust.

Hazards

If good working practices are observed then the service personnel are not exposed to any special biological hazards. Be careful to follow the manufacturer's procedure when lighting and turning off the flame.

Tools

A general tool kit is satisfactory.

Spares

Atomizer
Capillary tubing (plastic)
Capillary tube (metal)
Wire for cleaning capillary tubes
Gas cylinder
Photocell
Bulbs (when fitted)
Glass chimney (when fitted)

Maintenance

1. Remove the atomizer from the instrument and flush water through it.
2. Clean the metal capillary tube with thin wire to remove fibrin, dried serum, or plasma. Flush with water again.
3. If there is a built-in diluting pump, check the condition of the pump tubes and replace if necessary. Check that the dilution is correct (approximately) by preparing a calibrator, appropriately diluted using volumetric glassware, and comparing it with the dilution prepared by the pump. When the display is erratic, a volumetrically diluted calibrant will help to differentiate between a faulty pump and nebulizer/flame stability problems.

Service

1. Clean lenses, filters, and mirrors (if fitted) with a soft cloth to remove dust or carbon.
2. Clean the photocell with a soft cloth.
3. Clean the glass chimney.
4. Atomizers made of acrylic resin should be inspected for cracks. Replace as necessary.

Repair

Poor response may indicate a faulty photocell. If other possible causes have been eliminated (blocked atomizer, failed dilutor, old tubes, faulty power connections), then replace the photocell.

Calibration

Flame emission photometry is a comparative technique; therefore calibrators must be prepared and assayed simultaneously with the samples.

Gas cylinders and gases

It is assumed that hospital laboratories, theatres, and other departments that use gas cylinders will be using cylinders owned by the vendor. The problems of refilling will therefore not be considered. Cylinders are intrinsically simple devices (Fig. 2.17) requiring little or no maintenance. However, they are potentially highly dangerous because of the pressure of the contained gas. The pressure within a fully charged cylinder may be governed by local requirements, but can be as high as 20 MPa. For this reason, cylinders should be treated and maintained with care to avoid damage.

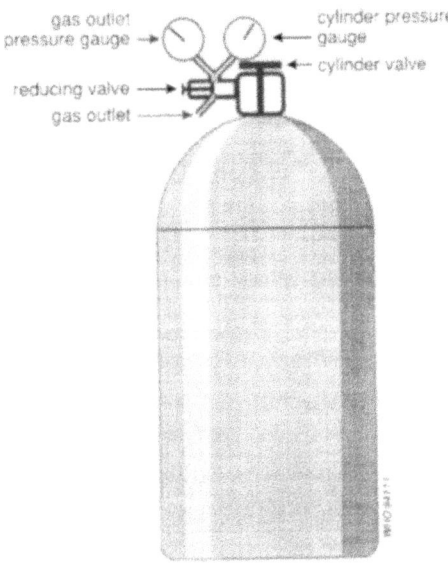

Fig. 2.17. Gas cylinder assembly.

Many gases are flammable, giving rise to an additional hazard. Even "harmless" gases, such as carbon dioxide and nitrogen, are potentially dangerous if allowed to escape into the atmosphere in high concentration, as they can cause asphyxiation by oxygen deprivation.

Gases, such as butane, that are liquid under storage conditions will exert vapour pressure within the cylinders all the time there is liquid present.

Procedures for the safe use and maintenance of cylinders

The name of the gas should be stamped or stencilled on the cylinder. Colour coding is also used for identification, but this may vary from country to country.

Labelling of cylinder caps is not acceptable as a means of identification, as these are interchangeable.

Cylinders should be kept in a purpose-built store and the gas piped to the area of utilization. Gas lines should be of an appropriate material for the safe distribution of the gas. Brass and steel pipes and fittings should **never** be connected together, since accelerated oxidation of the metals will occur, causing leaks. The lines should be clearly labelled.

Cylinders should not be subjected to extreme temperatures. (It is especially important that those containing flammable gases are not exposed to high temperatures.) This must be borne in mind when selecting the sites for gas stores.

Incompatible gases should not be stored together. Flammable gases (e.g., hydrogen, propane, butane) should not be stored with non-flammable gases (carbon dioxide, nitrogen, oxygen).

If a dedicated gas store is not available, and cylinders have to be stored in the working area, they must be fastened to the wall or bench with purpose-designed clamps. Flat-bottomed cylinders should not be used or stored free-standing, and purpose-designed or innovative stands should not be used as an alternative to clamping. Cylinders must be stored in a cool area away from sunlight. Oxygen cylinders used on the wards and other public areas should always be kept in a cylinder carrier.

Cylinders should never be emptied to below a pressure of 170 kPa. Empty cylinders should be clearly marked.

The main valve on an empty cylinder should not be left open. This will enable moisture to enter the cylinder, ultimately causing corrosion. It will also allow air to enter, which could create an explosive mixture with some flammable gases when the cylinder is refilled.

Cylinders must be fitted with the correct reducing-valve equipment. The operator must be familiar with the manufacturer's recommendations and adhere to these. Valve equipment should fit easily on to the cylinder, and should never be forced. If force is required, the fitting is probably inappropriate. Force may damage the valve and the cylinder.

Whenever a gas cylinder is to be connected to a regulator or piping system, the cylinder valve should be quickly "cracked" open and reclosed, in order to clear any debris accumulated in the valve outlet. Failure to do this can lead to plugged regulating valves and other disturbances. The cylinder should be clamped to the wall or bench before "cracking".

Separate reducing-valve equipment is required for flammable and non-flammable gases. These are specially designed, usually with a right-hand thread for non-flammable gases and a left-hand thread for flammable gases. However, this is not always the case, and the operator needs to be familiar with the manufacturer's practice and local requirements.

Reducing valves should always be used on cylinders that have a pressure greater than 700 kPa when full. Careful attention should be paid to the units on the manometer. Otherwise, misreading may lead to inappropriate handling of a gas cylinder.

The main cylinder valve should be opened slowly to avoid damaging the reducing valve. It should never be necessary to open the main valve fully, except with cylinders that are designed to operate with the valve fully open.

Oil should never be used to lubricate reducing valves, or any other part of the system.[1]

Only those tools provided, or recommended, by the manufacturer should be used for opening and shutting the main valve and for fitting or removing reducing valves. Undue force should not be required, as it is likely to damage the cylinder or the valve.

Cylinders should be transported with care to avoid fracture. They should not be dropped or rolled, and should be transported in an upright position on purpose-designed trolleys.

The operator must ensure that the cylinder and gas lines are leakproof. A leak of flammable gas is potentially explosive. Gases, such as hydrogen, that have a high diffusion rate, will escape from connections that would be leakproof for more dense gases. Connections should be checked regularly by dispensing a dilute soap solution on the fitting. A leak is indicated by the formation of bubbles.

Special requirements for the use of hazardous gases

As a general rule, it is strictly forbidden to smoke in the vicinity of gas cylinders.

Oxygen

Oxygen (O_2) is a normal constituent of the atmosphere, comprising 20–21% by volume. Oxygen is not flammable, but supports combustion, and in high oxygen concentrations almost everything will burn.

Valves, plumbing, and all fitments of oxygen gas cylinders must be scrupulously cleaned to remove all traces of organic material. Even new piping must be thoroughly cleaned before use. No equipment that is to be used in connection with oxygen should be touched with oily hands or gloves. Systems used for oxygen should never be used for any other gas.

Cylinders must be stored away from any combustible material.

Hydrogen

Hydrogen (H_2) is the lightest known gas, and therefore has a high diffusion rate. It will burn in oxygen in almost any concentration ratio, with a non-luminous flame which makes it difficult to see. It is fast burning, and fire spreads rapidly. Hydrogen is unique in that its temperature increases on expansion, with the risk of self-ignition if it is released too quickly from the cylinder. The main valve and reducing valve of a hydrogen gas cylinder should be opened slowly to avoid self-ignition.

All systems using hydrogen should be checked especially carefully for leaks.

Carbon dioxide

Carbon dioxide (CO_2) is a colourless, odourless, non-combustible, water-soluble gas. It is available in the form of a compressed liquid in gas cylinders, and in solid

---

[1] See also the recommendations for anaesthetic equipment, pp. 70–100.

form (dry ice). In the laboratory, it is used for the incubation of certain microbes, in the measurement of blood gases, and for other scientific purposes. In medicine, it is used as a respiratory stimulant. The liquid form is used in fire-extinguishers. Solid CO_2 is used primarily as a temporary laboratory coolant.

Carbon dioxide can accumulate at high concentrations in closed compartments, such as in closed rooms that are used for fermentation processes, or in wells, silos, mines, etc., where it diffuses to the bottom since it is more dense than air. A concentration of 5% carbon dioxide in the air will produce headaches and shortness of breath. A concentration of more than 10% can produce unconsciousness and death from oxygen deficiency. Such hazards can be easily avoided by appropriate room ventilation.

Nitrogen

Nitrogen (N_2) is the main component of air, comprising 78–79% by volume. It does not support the chemical reactions needed to maintain life. It can cause medical problems by displacing oxygen, leading to hypoxic asphyxia.

Compressed nitrogen is provided in gas cylinders, and is generally used in combination with oxygen gas, for better control of burning processes. In medicine, liquid nitrogen, which has a temperature of $-195\ °C$, is used for quick freezing and storage of tissues and microorganisms.

Nitrous oxide/oxygen mixtures

A 50/50 mixture of nitrous oxide and oxygen (N_2O/O_2) is often used for anaesthesia. If cylinders containing a nitrous oxide/oxygen mixture are stored at temperatures below 10 °C, the nitrous oxide can separate out. Therefore, the bottles must be warmed and shaken before use. Otherwise, the oxygen will be used first resulting in very high concentrations of nitrous oxide being delivered at a later stage, which will be hazardous to the patient.

Butane/propane

Butane (C_4H_6) and propane (C_3H_8) are colourless, odourless, flammable gases, and are usually mixed with foul-smelling additives to permit recognition of their presence. Although no special precautions are required in handling, the operator must be aware of their flammability. They are often supplied in small cylinders designed to fit on the back of analytical equipment. It must be remembered that, even in this quantity, these gases are explosive and potentially dangerous.

Butane and propane are stored as liquids under pressure. Therefore, cylinders must be kept upright, to prevent the liquids being forced into the piping system. In the laboratory, butane and propane are used for flame photometry.

Acetylene

Acetylene (C_2H_2) is a colourless gas with a faint ethereal odour. It is the most unstable compound any hospital worker is likely to encounter. Acetylene is used for atomic absorption spectroscopy, and also for the brazing, welding, cutting, and heating of metals. It will ignite explosively in air, over a wide concentration range. It is stabilized by the presence of certain other organic compounds, and is usually dissolved in acetone in commercially available cylinders. Acetylene reacts with many metals including copper, silver, and lead to form explosive acetylides.

Metal gas lines should not be used for acetylene, except at the express recommendation of the gas supplier. Stainless steel is acceptable, whereas copper pipes and soldered joints are not. Narrow-bore lines should be used, as acetylene is less stable in wide-bore pipes.

Operating gas pressure should not exceed 100 kPa. Only reducing valves that are specifically approved for acetylene should be used.

Special care must be taken with the storage and transportation of cylinders.

Acetylene is so dangerous that it should not be used in the hospital environment unless there is no alternative available.

Anaesthetic gases

There is no common standard for the identification of anaesthetic gas cylinders. For example, in North America, oxygen cylinders are usually green, those in Commonwealth countries are black with white shoulders, whereas in Switzerland and in France the cylinders are blue. Gas should not be administered to the patient unless the anaesthetist is absolutely certain of the contents of the cylinders.

When anaesthetic vapours are present in the operating room there is a risk of fire or explosion. It is important to distinguish between gas mixtures that are flammable and those that are explosive; the latter are much more dangerous to both staff and patients.

- Ether can be either flammable or explosive in the concentrations used for clinical purposes.
- 10% trichloroethylene will burn in oxygen.
- Mixtures of ether and air are flammable.
- Mixtures of ether and oxygen (or ether and nitrous oxide) are explosive.
- Oxygen and mixtures of oxygen and air are explosive.

There is a potential risk of explosion if diathermy equipment or other electrical apparatus is used in conjunction with flammable anaesthetic gases. Static electricity may also trigger an explosion if explosive gas mixtures are present. No potential source of combustion or electrical discharge should be allowed within 50 cm of an expiratory valve through which an explosive gas mixture is passing (e.g., ether/oxygen). Diathermy should be avoided altogether if a flammable gas mixture is in use, and vice versa.

Precautions

- The operating room and equipment should be rendered anti-static (it is worth remembering that moisture gives anti-static protection).
- Electrical sockets and switches should be either spark-proof, or situated at least 1 metre above floor level.
- The patient's expired gases should be carried away from the expiratory valve down a wide-bore tube at least to the floor (ether is heavier than air), or out of the operating room. Ensure that the tube is not kinked or blocked, and that there are no fire sources near its exit point.

Microscopes

Microscopes are used in medical laboratories to magnify images of light-transmitting or light-reflecting specimens. There are two main types of microscope: light microscopes and electron microscopes.

Light microscopes use glass optics to achieve magnification, while electron microscopes use electron beams and cathode ray tubes. For normal laboratory work, light microscopes are sufficient. Their maximum magnification power is usually 1000 times (microscope magnification = magnification of objective × magnification of eyepiece). A built-in electrical illuminator or a mirror to reflect artificial light or sunlight onto or through the specimen is used as a light source.

The light microscope is one of the most important instruments for laboratories in primary health care. The microscope needs daily attention to ensure reliable laboratory results.

Microscopes have the following components (Fig. 2.18):

- Stand: tube, tube support, base (foot), and stage.
- Optical system: objectives and eyepiece.
- Illumination system: light source (mirror or light bulb), condenser, and iris diaphragm.

Fig. 2.18. Light microscope.

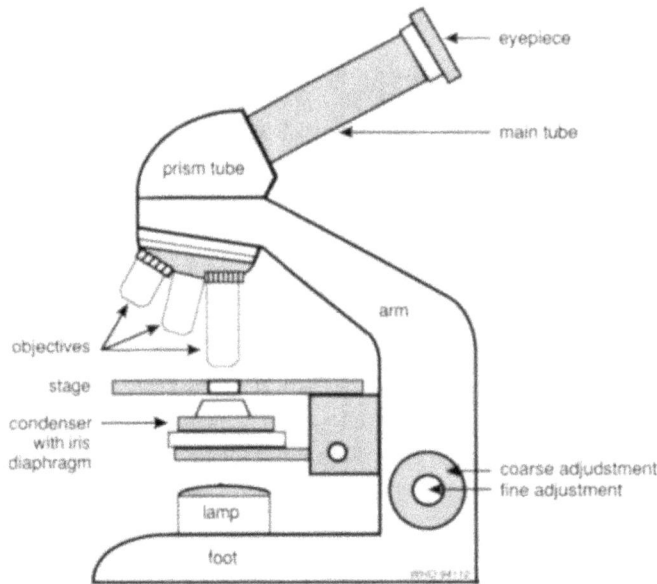

Installation

Microscopes must be installed in a clean environment, away from chemicals. Workplaces should be well ventilated or permanently air-conditioned (intermittent use of air-conditioners results in condensation). Humidity and higher temperatures often result in the growth of a fungus that can corrode optical surfaces. Optical instruments should not be kept for long periods in closed compartments since these conditions encourage fungal growth.

Cleaning of optics

Optical surfaces (condenser, objectives, eyepieces) must be kept free of dust with a soft camel hair brush or a blower. If dust is found inside the eyepiece, unscrew the upper lens and clean the inside with the blower or the soft brush.

Oil residues on the lenses should be removed with lens paper or absorbent paper or medical cotton wool. The optics may be finally cleaned with a special solution, consisting of 40% petroleum ether, 40% ethanol, and 20% ether.

Ethanol (96%) must not be used for cleaning the lenses, since it dissolves the cement. However, it can be used for cleaning mirrors.

Cleaning of instrument

Heavy contamination can be removed with mild soap solutions. Grease and oil can be removed with petroleum ether. The instrument should then be cleaned with a 50/50 mixture of distilled water and 96% ethanol. This solution is *not* suitable for cleaning the optics.

The mechanical parts (coarse adjustment, fine adjustment, condenser focusing, and mechanical stage) should be periodically cleaned and lubricated with a drop of machine oil to make them run freely.

Additional precautions to be taken in hot climates

Dry climates

In hot dry climates the main problem is dust. Fine particles work their way into the threads of the screws and under the lenses. This can be avoided as follows:

- Always keep the microscope under an air-tight plastic cover when not in use.
- At the end of the day's work, clean the microscope thoroughly by blowing air over it with a rubber bulb.
- Finish cleaning the lenses with a lens brush or fine paintbrush. If dust particles remain on the surface of the objective, clean it with lens paper.
- If there is a wet season lasting more than a month, take the precautions recommended below for hot humid climates.

Humid climates

In hot humid climates, fungus may develop on the microscope, particularly on the surface of the lenses, in the grooves of the screws, and under the paint, and the instrument will soon be useless. This can be prevented as described below.

Always keep the microscope under an air-tight plastic cover when not in use, with a dish filled with blue silica to desiccate the air under the cover. (The silica will turn red when it has lost its capacity to absorb moisture from the air. It can be simply regenerated by heating in a hot air oven or over a fire.) The microscope must be cleaned daily to get rid of dust.

Use and maintenance[1]

- Never dip the objectives in xylene or ethanol (the lenses would become unstuck).

---

[1] More details and useful advice are given in the document, *Function, use and maintenance of routine microscopes*, obtainable from Health Laboratory Technology and Blood Safety, World Health Organization, 1211 Geneva 27, Switzerland. (This document was prepared by the Zeiss company, and supplied to WHO for free distribution.)

- Never use ordinary paper to clean the lenses.
- Never touch the lenses with your fingers.
- Never clean the supports or the stage with xylene or acetone.
- Never clean the inside lenses of the eyepieces and objectives with cloth or paper (this might remove the anti-reflective coating); use a fine paintbrush only.
- Never leave the microscope without the eyepieces unless the openings are plugged.
- Never keep the microscope in a closed wooden box in hot humid countries.
- Never press the objective onto the slide, since both slide and objective may break. Take care when focusing the microscope.
- Keep the mechanical stage clean.
- Do not dismantle the optical components, as this may cause misalignment. The optics should be cleaned by using lens-cleaning tissue or soft toilet paper.
- Never put the microscope away with immersion oil on the objective. Remove any oil daily. Mild soap solution is suitable for most cleaning.
- Organic solvents should only be used in accordance with the manufacturer's recommendations.
- When changing a bulb, avoid touching the glass with the fingers, as fingerprints reduce the intensity of illumination.
- The life-span of bulbs is extended considerably by adjusting voltage to give the lowest required light intensity.
- If the mains voltage fluctuates excessively, use a voltage stabilizer.

Repairs

In all repair and maintenance procedures, care must be taken not to confuse the condenser centring screws with the condenser clamp screws.

1. Check mechanical stage.
2. Check focusing mechanism.
3. Remove fungal growth.
4. Check diaphragms.
5. Clean mechanical parts.
6. Lubricate to manufacturer's specification.
7. Check spring load on specimen clamp. Too high a tension may result in breakage of slides and damage to clamp.
8. Check optical alignment. Dim appearance of the specimen is often due to misalignment of the optics rather than to insufficient light.

Hazards

As microscopes are used to investigate biological tissues and fluids, they must be decontaminated at regular intervals. The mechanical parts may be decontaminated with 70% ethanol, and the optical parts should be cleaned according to the manufacturer's instructions. These procedures must be carried out regularly, and are essential in conjunction with repair and maintenance procedures.

Tools

Rubber-bulb blower
Paintbrush (fine and soft)

Spares

Bulbs
Racks

Pinions, suitable ball and roller bearings
Eyepieces (must be stored under dry and dust-free conditions)
Objectives (must be stored under dry and dust-free conditions)
Greases, oils (see manufacturer's recommendations)
Fungal cleaning solution
Illumination mirror

Photometers

A photometer is an optical instrument that is used to measure absorption of light. According to the Lambert–Beer Law, the absorption of light by a solution is related to the concentration of the solute. The photometer is an essential instrument for a laboratory, and can be used for the determination of a great number of analytes in body fluids. Photometers differ as regards their light source and the way in which the monochromatic light is generated. The following types are found:

- Instrument with a light source that emits a spectrum of discrete lines (cadmium or mercury lamp).
- Instrument with a source that generates a continuous spectrum of light (white light) (tungsten–halogen lamp), which is split by a prism or a grating into its different components.
- Instrument with a source that emits a continuous spectrum of light (tungsten–halogen lamp) which is filtered to produce light with a desired wavelength.
- Instrument with a diode lamp that emits monochromatic light.

The instruments may be of the single- or double-beam type. In a single-beam instrument, light passes from the source through a monochromator or filter and then via a sample cuvette to the detector. In a double-beam instrument, light passes through a beam-splitting device and then via separate sample and reference cuvettes to separate detectors.

The instruments with a tungsten light source and filters are usually referred to as photometers, or in a simpler version as colorimeters; the more complex instruments with interference filters, prisms or gratings are referred to as spectrometers.

The essential elements of a photometer or spectrometer are shown in Fig. 2.19.

Fig. 2.19. Photometer assembly.

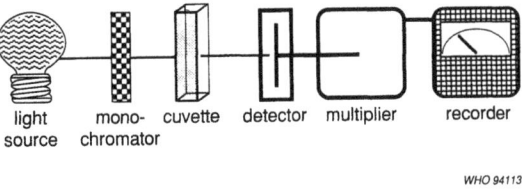

The positions of the monochromator and the cuvette are reversed in certain instruments. All of these elements are prone to defects. The diode-lamp photometer does not need a filter or prism since the emitted light is already monochromatic.

Light source

The light source in a photometer may generate either light with a continuous spectrum of wavelengths (tungsten lamp), light with a discrete spectrum of wavelengths (mercury lamp) or monochromatic light (light-emitting diode). To cover the entire range of wavelengths, spectrometers generally have two lamps, one generating light in the ultraviolet range (200–400 nm) and the other generating light in the visible range (400–800 nm) (Fig. 2.20).

Fig. 2.20. Spectra of the light emitted by spectrometer bulbs.

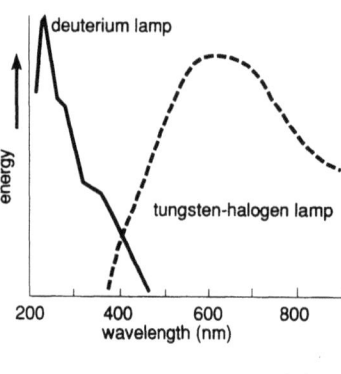

Lamps are prone to slow but continuous attrition, and need to be checked periodically. If the lamp is the cause of instability of the absorption signal, it should be replaced. After a new lamp has been fitted, the optics of the system should be realigned as follows, to ensure that the maximum amount of light reaches the photocell after passing through the cuvette.

1. Place a cuvette filled with distilled water, and a filter, in position.
2. Set the meter to a mid-scale reading, roughly 0.3 (50% transmission).
3. Move each optical component, in turn, very slightly, and check whether the reading is affected.
4. If necessary, adjust the lamp alignment to obtain maximum transmission.

In some instruments, it is possible to place a white card immediately in front of the photocell. A clear image of the lamp filament should be seen on the card. If the image is out of focus, or not vertical, the lamp alignment should be adjusted until the best image is obtained.

Monochromators

Monochromators are used to disperse the white light into its different light components, one of which is selected for photometric measurement. Two types of monochromator exist: the prism and the grating (Fig. 2.21).

Fig. 2.21. Dispersion of white light by (a) a prism, (b) a transmission grating.

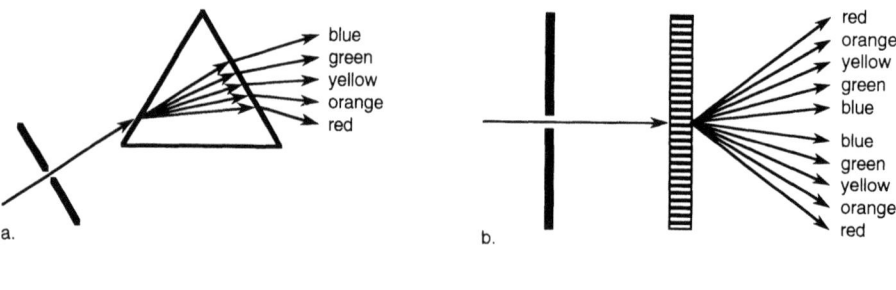

In spectrometers, the monochromator must be correctly aligned. This can be checked by observing the absorbance maxima of a known reference solution, or reference absorbing material. Table 2.9 shows the specific absorbance values of a potassium dichromate solution (60 mg in 1 litre of 0.005 mol/litre aqueous sulfuric acid).

Table 2.9. **Specific absorbance values of a standard potassium dichromate solution**

Wavelength (nm)	Specific absorbance (A_1^1)[a]
235	124.5 (±1.6)
257	144.0 (±1.6)
313	48.6 (±1.6)
350	106.6 (±1.6)

[a] The specific absorbance (A_1^1) is defined as the absorbance of a 1% (10 g/litre) solution of the solute in a cell with 1 cm path-length.

A holmium oxide glass filter can also be used as a reference absorbing material; it has major peaks at the following wavelengths: 241.5 nm, 279.4 nm, 287.5 nm, 333.7 nm, 360.9 nm, 418.4 nm, 453.2 nm, 536.2 nm, and 637.5 nm.

Filters

Filters absorb light of different wavelengths, allowing only light with a narrow range of wavelengths (band width) to pass through. Filters for a photometer have a band width of about 2 nm, while filters for a colorimeter are of lower quality and have a wider band width (20–40 nm). Thus more light will pass through the filter of a colorimeter and the same sample solution will give a higher reading than in a photometer. The difference in the quality of filters explains why a colorimeter is less sensitive than a photometer, and why the calibration factor for measurement with a colorimeter is higher than that for a standardized measurement with a photometer. Calibration factors for a specific method, using a specific reagent, may be given by the manufacturer or may be found in the literature. However, calibration factors are usually only valid when the measurement is made at the specified wavelength in a photometer with narrow band width. The calibration factor must be determined separately when measurement is made in a colorimeter, or when measurements are compared with a calibration curve produced from a different instrument and with a different filter.

Filters may be fixed or removable. If the filters can be removed, they should not be left in the photometer when it is not in use, but should be stored in a dust-free box to ensure that they cannot be broken. They should be fitted into position before the lamp is switched on so that the photocell is not damaged.

Cuvettes

A cuvette is the transparent container used to hold the test solution. Cuvettes may be made out of quartz glass, normal glass, or transparent plastic, such as polystyrene or polyamide. Most cuvettes are rectangular, with an internal pathway of exactly 1 cm. Occasionally, they are cylindrical. Cuvettes made out of quartz glass may be used with light sources producing visible (wavelength 400–800 nm) or ultraviolet (200–400 nm) light. Normal glass and plastic cuvettes may be used with light of wavelength between 340 nm (preferably 365 nm) and 800 nm, and are suitable for routine measurements. Plastic cuvettes are usually of poorer quality, but they are cheaper than glass cuvettes and can be discarded after use. On the other hand, glass cuvettes are easier to clean for re-use, and do not deteriorate if properly handled.

The cuvettes must be scrupulously clean if accurate measurements are to be obtained. Precipitates on glass cuvettes from protein solutions may be removed by soaking overnight in a concentrated sulfuric acid/potassium dichromate solution. Subsequently, they must be thoroughly rinsed with distilled water and left to dry inverted on a clean piece of absorbent paper. Plastic cuvettes must not be cleaned in strong acid; use a detergent solution. These solutions, however, leave a film on the cuvette resulting in an increased absorbance. Cuvettes should be stored in a dust-free box to prevent scratching.

Remember, the following errors will lead to incorrect measurements:

- incorrect size of cuvette,
- scratched cuvettes,
- damaged cuvettes,
- incorrect positioning of the cuvette.

Detector and multiplier

The detector and multiplier are electronic components that may fail as a result of aging, careless handling of the instrument, or incorrect connection to the electrical power supply. Faults in the monochromator system or photocell and multiplier system may be the cause of deviations from linearity in measurements of a dilution series. Deviations from linearity are also caused by high concentrations of an absorbent in the solution. Therefore, the correct functioning of a photometer needs to be checked periodically with special control solutions, such as acid potassium dichromate.

The absence of a display response can indicate breakdown of the detector. This can be confirmed if light can be seen on a white card held in front of the detector. A new photocell is then required.

Photometric measurement

The relationship between the intensity of light entering and leaving a cuvette filled with a solution that absorbs light of a given wavelength is described by the Lambert–Beer law. The fraction of the incident light absorbed is proportional to the number of solute molecules in the light path, i.e.,

$$\log \frac{I_o}{I} = k \times c \times b$$

where I_o = incident light intensity,
I = transmitted light intensity,
c = solute concentration (mol/l),
b = path length (cm),
k = calibration coefficient.

The absorbance is defined as the logarithm of the ratio I_o/I. Theoretically the absorbance of light may vary from zero (no absorbance) to infinity (complete absorbance). A photometer is most accurate in the absorbance range between 0 and 1.0, and in good instruments up to 2.0. With a colorimeter, reliable results are obtained between 0 and 0.7.

The constant k is a fundamental property of the solute, and is dependent on temperature, wavelength, and solvent.

All the cuvettes used for measurement and calibration must have the same absorbance. As a check, all cuvettes to be used for measurement should be filled with distilled water and placed into the cuvette holder. After zeroing the instrument, measure the absorbance of each cuvette; the absorbance should not exceed 0.01. Cuvettes with a higher absorbance must not be used, or must be matched with other cuvettes having the same absorbance to eliminate "cuvette error".

The use of a single cuvette for all the measurements on a series of specimens avoids "cuvette error". Fill the cuvette with a blank solution appropriate to the type of test, and set the instrument to zero using this blank. Then discard the blank solution, turn the cuvette upside down and shake it to remove the last drops of the blank solution prior to refilling with the first test solution. The level of the solution in the cuvette must be high enough to ensure that reflection of light from the surface does not interfere with the measurement of absorbance. Also, any air bubbles trapped against the walls of the cuvette must be removed by gently tapping the cuvette with the finger.

A major source of error in photometric measurement is drift of the zero setting during determination of a series of specimens. To avoid errors, the zero should be readjusted after each 5 or 10 measurements, by measuring the light absorption by a cuvette filled with distilled water or reagent solution. Never check the zero with an empty cuvette.

Light absorption is measured in specimens diluted with buffer and with reagent solution for reaction. All solutions, i.e., the specimen, the buffer, the reagent solution, and the final mixture after incubation, should be clear. If the final solution is turbid, the transparency of the cuvette must be checked and the investigation repeated.

The presence of stray light can be determined by measuring the light absorbance by a substance that has infinite absorbance at that wavelength. The following solutions/liquids have infinite absorbance over the stated wavelength ranges, and are suitable for measuring stray light:

aqueous potassium chloride (12 g/l)	175–200 nm
aqueous sodium bromide (10 g/l)	195–223 nm
aqueous sodium iodide (10 g/l)	210–259 nm
acetone	250–320 nm
aqueous sodium nitrite (50 g/l)	300–385 nm

Set the spectrometer at the wavelength to be checked for stray light. Select an appropriate solution or liquid. Adjust the instrument to infinite absorbance. Change the wavelength setting to a longer wavelength and set to zero absorbance. Return to the original wavelength setting and measure the absorbance. Any reading less than infinity is due to stray light.

Remember:

- Never use a cuvette without having run a blank determination. It is possible that at high concentrations of the analyte the limits for linear measurement are exceeded.
- When the reaction time in a cuvette is prolonged, the cuvette should be sealed to avoid evaporation of the solvent; otherwise, the concentration of the analyte will increase and result in higher light absorption.
- Cuvettes have two optical walls, where the light beam passes through, and two non-optical walls. They should be held only by the non-optical walls.

- The surface of the solution to be measured in the cuvette must be above the height of the light beam passing through the cuvette; otherwise, light scattering at the surface of the liquid may change the magnitude of the absorption signal.
- When using semi-micro and micro cuvettes, they must be correctly positioned in the light path, otherwise light will be partially reflected and a false reading will be obtained.

Comparators

These are portable devices in which the intensity of colour developed in a solution of unknown concentration is visually compared with that of a known concentration. A good source of natural light is required in order to carry out the colour matching.

When not in use, store the comparator and the standard filter discs in a dark, dust-free container.

Unpacking, siting, installation

Unpack the instrument carefully, and assemble according to the instruction manual supplied. Keep specialized packaging for possible future use.

Set the instrument on a firm and level bench that is free from vibration and away from any strong lighting (especially sunlight). The environment should be free of dust, fumes and smoke. Tobacco smoke can be a serious cause of deteriorating optical performance.

Check that the voltage and fuse rating are in accordance with the manufacturer's instructions.

Good practice

- Handle optical components only by the sides, to avoid contamination.
- Use of clean and matched cuvettes is vital if the full performance of photometers and comparators is to be realized.
- Occasionally soak the cuvettes in mild detergent for a few hours. Rinse thoroughly with distilled water and invert to dry.
- Store cuvettes in a dust-free box, and ensure that they cannot scratch each other by contact.
- For filter photometers and comparators, keep spare filters in a dust-free box, and ensure they cannot be broken or scratched.
- Any spillages on or around the instrument should be cleaned up immediately.
- Turn off the lamp after use, to ensure maximum life.
- Do not leave cuvettes in the instrument.
- Ensure that a filter is in position (in filter photometers) when the lamp is turned on, to avoid damaging the photocell.

Hazards

If good working practices are observed, there are no special precautions.

Special tools/requirements/spares

A general tool kit and lens tissues are required.

Spares: source lamps
　　　　fuses
　　　　cuvettes
　　　　photocell

A calibrating filter is required to check the wavelength accuracy of spectrometers.

Maintenance

When the instrument is cool, and with the electricity turned off:

1. Clean the filters and optical windows with lens tissue.
2. Keep the cuvettes clean (see page 44).

Service

The window and/or front surface of the photodetector should be inspected periodically, and cleaned with lens tissues.

Check lamp alignment (see page 42).

Wavelength calibration (spectrometers only)

By inserting a calibrating filter in the cuvette compartment in place of a normal cuvette, the wavelength calibration may be checked as follows:

1. Turn the wavelength control slowly and identify the peaks described in the data sheet accompanying the filter.
2. If the instrument is more than 5 nm off calibration, apply the manufacturer's instructions for recalibration.

Repair

1. If there is no display response, but light is passing through the system, then change the photocell.
2. If there is no light passing through the system change the lamp. This may also be necessary if the light signal does not remain constant during measurement (as indicated by unreproducible results of extinction obtained from repeated measurements using the same cuvette).

Pipettes, autopipettes, and dispensers

Pipettes are instruments that are used for transferring a predetermined volume of liquid from one vessel to another. They are not connected to a reservoir. There are so many types of pipette that it is difficult to discuss the subject systematically. It should be noted that the replacement of broken conventional calibrated pipettes is often very costly, and that it may be cheaper in the long run to use mechanical pipettes.

Fig. 2.22. A mechanical micropipette.

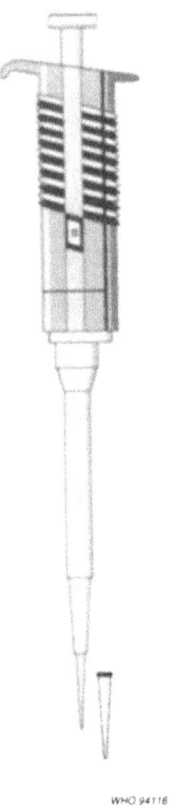

Mechanical pipettes

Mechanical micropipettes (Fig. 2.22) can only be recommended where a reliable supply of new disposable tips is readily available. They are used for the delivery and/or dilution of biological samples in the volume range 5–1000 µl. They are usually of air displacement (indirect) or direct displacement design. To avoid contamination between consecutive samples, most pipettes have a disposable tip that is discarded after each delivery. This greatly increases the cost per test. The practice of washing and reusing disposable tips is not recommended, as any cleaning procedures will change the "wettability" of the plastic. In addition, drying at only slightly elevated temperatures may distort the tip, and prevent a good pneumatic seal with the pipette body.

Alternative sample pipettes

Any system that requires mouth-pipetting of biological samples is unacceptable because of the high risk of infection from accidental aspiration of contaminated material. Thus, the traditional shell-backed pipettes used with a haemocytometer-type tube and mouthpiece should never be used.

Sanz pipettes

A pipette that meets the requirements of safe handling and precision is the Sanz pipette. It is available in two forms; one is for the accurate measurement of samples (Fig. 2.23a), the other is for the repeated delivery of reagents in the range 5–100 µl (Fig. 2.23b).

Fig. 2.23. Sanz pipettes.

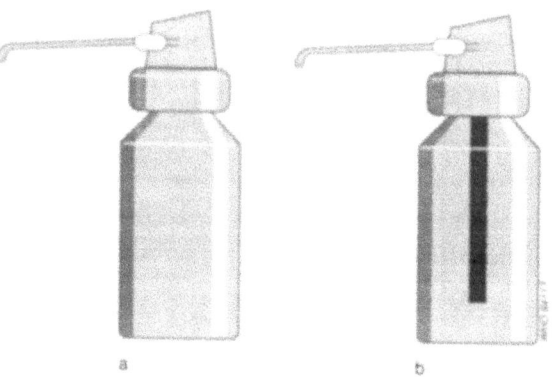

Sanz pipettes have a high precision (coefficient of variation: 0.5% in the range 5–100 µl), are very robust, and can be made locally.

Dispensers and dilutors

Dispensers are instruments for delivering predetermined volumes of liquid from a reservoir. The reservoir may be an integral part of the instrument, or connected externally. Dilutors are instruments for taking up different liquids (e.g., sample and diluent) and delivering them together in a predetermined ratio and/or predetermined volume. The reservoirs of the diluent may be an integral part of the instrument, or connected externally (Fig. 2.24).

Fig. 2.24. Diluter.

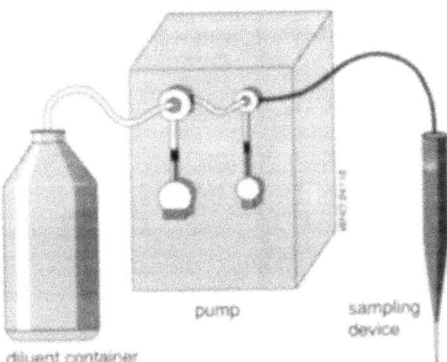

Maintenance and repair

It is virtually impossible to give helpful general advice on the maintenance and repair of dispensers and autopipettes because there are so many different types. The manufacturer's instructions and recommendations should be followed.

Pipetting

When the specimen is being mixed with a reagent and buffer solution, the appropriate pipette (or pipette tip) must be used for each individual step of the procedure. Pipetting by mouth should be forbidden because of the biological and chemical hazards. A small rubber bulb (Peleus ball) with two valves (Fig. 2.25) should be fixed to the top of the pipette. The pipette is held vertically while being filled by suction. The position of the bottom of the meniscus on the pipette scale indicates the exact volume (Fig. 2.26). When the solution is expelled, the pipette must also be held vertically. It should be kept in this position for 5 seconds after the outflow of the last drop. After use, semi-automated pipettes must be kept in an *upright* position and thoroughly cleaned periodically.

Fig. 2.26. Use of a glass pipette.

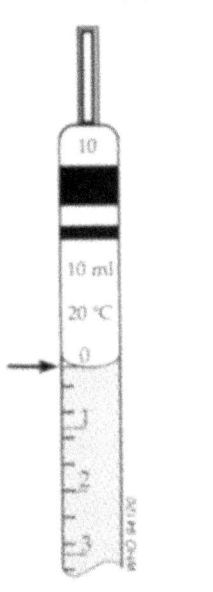

Fig. 2.25. Peleus ball.

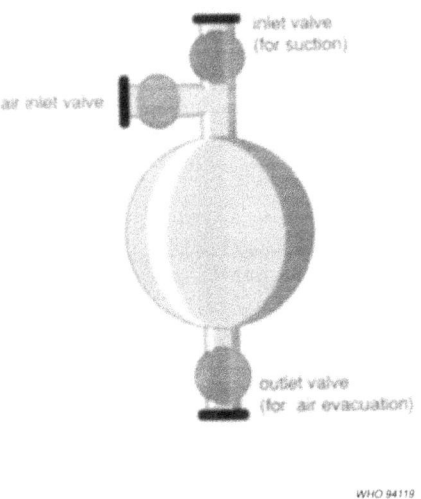

Semi-automated pipettes should be calibrated every 3 months, using appropriate dye solutions.

Plastic pipette tips must be tested for air-tightness. If there is not a good seal, the solution will leak out. Cheap pipette tips are often of poor quality, and therefore useless. A single pipette tip can be used for serial pipetting of a solution. Although the same tip may be used repeatedly for the same solution, it must be replaced before different solutions or samples are pipetted.

Testing and calibration

Requirements: distilled water
analytical balance
thermometer (readable to 0.1 °C)
barometer ($\pm$ 25 mbar)
weighing vessel (10–50 times the test volume, with cover or cap).

When verifying the performance of an instrument, pipetting must be repeated at least 10 times to estimate accuracy and at least 30 times to estimate within-run precision. For subsequent control evaluations, the estimate for within-run precision should be made after pipetting at least 10 times, and the estimate of accuracy after pipetting at least 4 times. The general procedure is based on gravimetric analysis of water samples delivered by the instrument. The values are corrected for evaporation. True mass and volume are then calculated simultaneously, based on the density of water at specific temperatures, and corrections for air buoyancy.

Note: For safety reasons the use of mercury for gravimetric calibration should be discouraged.

Procedure

1. Deliver a total of n samples into a covered weighing vessel and weigh each sample after delivery. Replicate as precisely as possible all motions and time intervals in each sampling cycle. Use a randomly selected pipette tip either only once for each sample weighing or repeatedly for the n weighings.
2. Measure a control blank by dispensing a pre-tared volume of water into the covered weighing vessel, to estimate the degree of evaporation under the experimental conditions. Then duplicate all motions and time intervals as in normal pipetting, with the exception that no more liquid is added to the weighing vessel. Use the resultant mean loss of weight as the correction value for evaporation.
3. Measure and record the temperature of the water to 0.1 °C, before and after the weighing procedure. The temperature (t) is the average of the two measurements of water temperature, rounded to the nearest 0.5 °C.

Calculations

Calculate the mean volume (V) delivered at the test temperature (t) from the mean weighing result (w) by adding the mean evaporation (e) and correcting the sum by an appropriate factor that allows for density and buoyancy corrections when water is weighed in air, at the test temperature and pressure, and standard humidity.

1. Calculate the individual weighing results (w_i) by subtracting the tare reading from the sample reading for each sample.
2. Calculate the mean weight ($\bar{w}$) from the individual weighings (w_i):

$$\bar{w} = \frac{\sum w_i}{n}$$

where n = number of samples.

3. Calculate the evaporation e from the number of determinations as follows:

$$e = \frac{\sum e_i}{n_e}$$

where e_i = individual determination and n_e = number of control blanks.

4. Calculate the mean volume of the liquid samples ($\bar{V}_t$) from the mean weight ($\bar{w}$):

$$\bar{V}_t = (\bar{w} + e) \times z$$

where z = conversion factor (μl/mg) at the test temperature and pressure. (Values of z for distilled water, at various test temperatures, are listed in Table 2.10.)

5. Calculate the percentage inaccuracy ($\bar{E}_t$) of the instrument at the test temperature (t) as the difference between the nominal volume of the instrument (V_o) and the calculated mean volume $\bar{V}_t$:

$$\bar{E}_t = \frac{\bar{V}_t - V_o}{V_o} \times 100$$

Table 2.10. Values for z (μl/mg), as a function of temperature and pressure, for distilled water

Temperature (°C)	Air pressure					
	600	640	680	720	760	800 (mmHg)
	800	853	907	960	1013	1067 (mbar)
	80.0	85.3	90.7	96.0	101.3	106.7 (kPa)
15	1.0018	1.0018	1.0019	1.0019	1.0020	1.0020
15.5	1.0018	1.0019	1.0019	1.0020	1.0020	1.0021
16	1.0019	1.0020	1.0020	1.0021	1.0021	1.0022
16.5	1.0020	1.0020	1.0021	1.0022	1.0022	1.0023
17	1.0021	1.0021	1.0022	1.0022	1.0023	1.0023
17.5	1.0022	1.0022	1.0023	1.0023	1.0024	1.0024
18	1.0022	1.0023	1.0024	1.0024	1.0025	1.0025
18.5	1.0023	1.0024	1.0025	1.0025	1.0026	1.0026
19	1.0024	1.0025	1.0025	1.0026	1.0027	1.0027
19.5	1.0025	1.0026	1.0026	1.0027	1.0028	1.0028
20	1.0026	1.0027	1.0027	1.0028	1.0029	1.0029
20.5	1.0027	1.0028	1.0028	1.0029	1.0030	1.0030
21	1.0028	1.0029	1.0030	1.0030	1.0031	1.0031
21.5	1.0030	1.0030	1.0031	1.0031	1.0032	1.0032
22	1.0031	1.0031	1.0032	1.0032	1.0033	1.0033
22.5	1.0032	1.0032	1.0033	1.0033	1.0034	1.0035
23	1.0033	1.0033	1.0034	1.0035	1.0035	1.0036
23.5	1.0034	1.0035	1.0035	1.0036	1.0036	1.0037
24	1.0035	1.0036	1.0036	1.0037	1.0038	1.0038
24.5	1.0037	1.0037	1.0038	1.0038	1.0039	1.0039
25	1.0038	1.0038	1.0039	1.0039	1.0040	1.0041
25.5	1.0039	1.0040	1.0040	1.0041	1.0041	1.0042
26	1.0040	1.0041	1.0042	1.0042	1.0043	1.0043
26.5	1.0042	1.0042	1.0043	1.0043	1.0044	1.0045
27	1.0043	1.0044	1.0044	1.0045	1.0045	1.0046
27.5	1.0044	1.0045	1.0046	1.0046	1.0047	1.0047
28	1.0046	1.0046	1.0047	1.0048	1.0048	1.0049
28.5	1.0047	1.0048	1.0048	1.0049	1.0050	1.0050
29	1.0049	1.0049	1.0050	1.0050	1.0051	1.0052
29.5	1.0050	1.0051	1.0051	1.0052	1.0052	1.0053
30	1.0052	1.0052	1.0053	1.0053	1.0054	1.0055

6. Calculate the within-run imprecision (coefficient of variation, CV) from the distribution of the individual weighings (w_i) about their mean ($\bar{w}$), corrected for error due to evaporation:

$$CV = \frac{100 \times s}{(\bar{w} + e)}$$

where $s = \frac{(w_i - \bar{w})^2}{n - 1}$

Refrigerators

Refrigeration is the result of the absorption of energy (heat) during the evaporation of a liquid. A refrigerant liquid is circulated through a closed system of pipes, in which on one side (refrigeration chamber) it is vaporized and on the other side (outside the refrigeration chamber) it is condensed. Common refrigerant liquids are ammonia (boiling point $-33\,°C$), and low relative molecular mass chlorofluorocarbons (boiling point near $-30\,°C$). The vaporization of the refrigerant liquid is achieved by either absorption or compression.

Absorption

The absorption system is used mainly in small refrigerators, because it requires more energy input than the compressor system. The closed system of an absorption refrigerator consists of an evaporator, an absorption vessel, a heating chamber and a condenser (Fig. 2.27). The liquid contains ammonia as refrigerant and water as absorbant. The third component in the system is hydrogen, which accelerates the evaporation of ammonia and maintains a constant pressure in the circuit.

Fig. 2.27. Working principle of an absorption refrigerator.

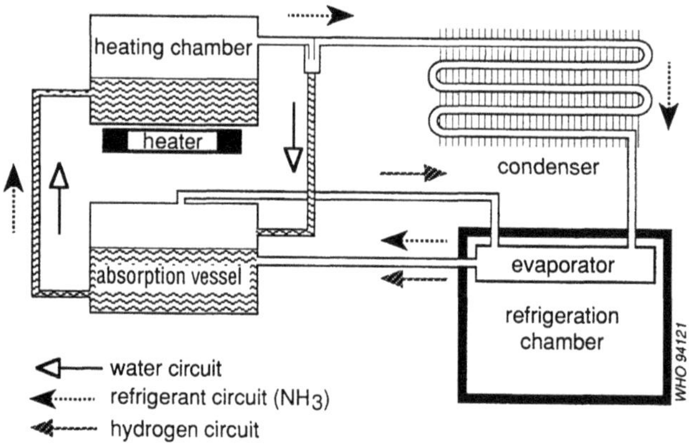

The circuit works at constant pressure and has no moving parts. The operation of the circuit is based on the following principles:

- Water can absorb large quantities of ammonia at ordinary temperatures. The absorption of ammonia in water occurs so fast that a "compression" effect results.
- At modestly elevated temperatures, ammonia separates from water into the gaseous phase.
- Hydrogen does not dissolve in water.

— The laws of partial pressure state that, in a space occupied by a mixture of gases that do not react chemically together, each gas exerts the pressure that it would produce if it occupied the space alone, and the total pressure is the sum of these pressures.

When a mixture of ammonia and water is heated by a flame or an electrical device in the heating chamber, ammonia and a relatively small amount of water will evaporate. The ammonia and water vapour enter a percolator, where the water is condensed. This water, containing a low concentration of ammonia, passes into the absorption vessel. The gaseous ammonia moves to the condenser. Air circulating over the fins of the condenser cools the gaseous ammonia, and it condenses. The liquid ammonia then flows by gravitational forces into the evaporator where it evaporates under low pressure at ambient temperature. This process extracts heat from the storage compartment. The evaporation is accelerated by hydrogen gas passing across the surface of the ammonia. The ammonia–hydrogen mixture travels to the absorption chamber, where the ammonia is absorbed by the water. This process occurs so fast that it keeps the partial pressure of ammonia in the system low and contributes to accelerating evaporation in the evaporator. The hydrogen passes through the water without being absorbed and back to the evaporator.

With the absorption of ammonia the liquid in the absorption chamber increases in density and flows into the heating chamber, from where the refrigeration cycle is repeated.

Compression

Compression systems are used for cold rooms and for some small refrigerators and require mains electricity. They consist of an evaporator, an expansion valve or capillary pipe, a condenser, and a compressor (Fig. 2.28).

Fig. 2.28. Working principle of a compression refrigerator.

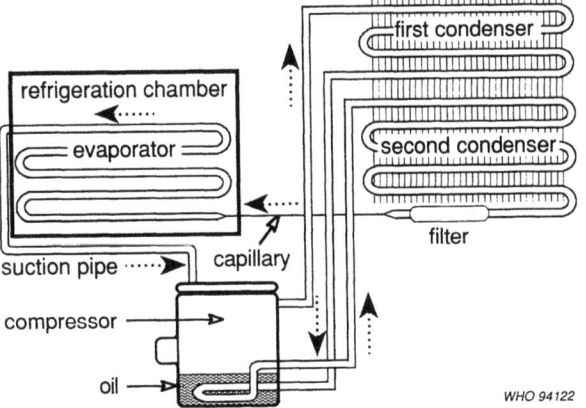

A compressor sucks the coolant liquid from the tubes of the evaporator, which are located inside the cooling compartment of the refrigerator. The residual coolant liquid in the evaporator evaporates and in doing so takes up latent heat from the cooling compartment. The vapour is compressed into pipes outside the refrigerator, where it condenses, liberating heat, which is dissipated to the surrounding air by the condenser fins. The condensed coolant liquid is forced through the capillary pipe and expands into the evaporator, from where the refrigeration cycle is repeated. In some refrigerators, the condensed coolant is circulated back to the compressor to take up heat from the compressor oil, which again causes evaporation of the refrigerant. In a second condenser, the coolant is condensed again prior to passing through the capillary tube for expansion and evaporation, while the liberated heat of condensation is dissipated to the environment.

Installation

Electrical compressor-operated refrigerators and freezers should be used only where there is a stable and reliable electricity supply. Fluctuations in the voltage, and frequent power interruptions, are likely to result in damage to the compressor. Absorption refrigerators and freezers are preferred in situations where electricity supply is unreliable.

Equipment should be installed on a flat, horizontal surface, preferably slightly elevated (on pallet or feet) to avoid accumulation of water and moisture under the cabinet. This will prevent the formation of rust and allow easy access for cleaning.

Good practice

- Keep the surrounding area clean.
- Leave at least 20 cm between the cabinet and the wall and other equipment, and avoid exposure to heat and sunshine.
- Keep the refrigerator upright and level. If the cabinet needs to be moved, it should be transported in an upright position.
- Wash the door gasket with soap solution, and rub with glycerol, when the cabinet is defrosted.
- Do not re-open the door immediately after closing.
- Never use sharp instruments to remove ice. Defrosting may be quickened by placing a container of warm water in the refrigerator or freezer after electrical isolation.
- Remove all water from the inside of the refrigerator or freezer after defrosting.
- Do not leave the refrigerator or freezer open unnecessarily.
- Open and close the door gently.

Flammable chemicals must only be stored in cabinets designed for that purpose. Kerosene-operated refrigerators and freezers should be refilled with uncontaminated kerosene. The burner, chimney, and wick must be cleaned regularly. The baffle must be inserted into the chimney.

Maintenance

The following general advice may be helpful for maintenance:

- The refrigerator must be placed so that sufficient air can flow past the condenser (at the back of the refrigerator) for exchange of heat.
- The refrigerator door must seal perfectly to prevent warm outside air from entering the cool chamber.
- The refrigerator must have good insulating walls.
- For photovoltaic (solar-powered) refrigerators, the collector must be positioned so as to receive maximum solar radiation; it must be cleaned periodically to ensure the production of enough electricity.

Daily checks

- Check temperature daily.
- Check the gas bottles or kerosene tank, in the case of gas or kerosene refrigerators, so that more can be ordered in good time.

Monthly checks

- Clear the cool chamber, and defrost the evaporator once a month.
- Swab inside the cabinet with 70% ethanol while it is defrosting.
- Clean the outside of the refrigerator.
- Clean any dust from the condenser.
- Clean the door gasket.
- Clean the burner, and check for gas leakage.
- In photovoltaic refrigerators, check the level of electrolyte solution in the batteries, and fill up with pure distilled water, if necessary.

Door gaskets

On domestic-type refrigerators, the gasket-holding mechanism is the inner shell of the door. This fastens to the outer casing with a ring of screws under the gasket. When this is disassembled in order to change the gasket, the rigidity of the door structure is lost. In order to ensure a good seal upon reassembly, the complete door must first be removed and placed on several boards to keep it as flat as possible. Then, remove the screws and the old gasket, install the new gasket and replace the screws before moving the door. Reinstall the door, with the hinge screws snug but not tight. Shut the door with a piece of paper in the seal, and test for tightness by pulling on the paper. Do this all around the gasket. The hinges may be adjusted outwards by closing the door with a folded cloth in the seal or by bumping with a soft rubber mallet. Adjust until the paper indicates that the door is evenly tight all around, then tighten the screws in the hinges.

Compressor-type refrigerators and freezers

- Clean the condenser (in the compressor compartment) every 6 months with a brush or vacuum cleaner.
- Oil the door fittings, locks, and other moving parts.
- Replacement of the compressor, which would require recharging with refrigerant, should be carried out only by a qualified refrigeration engineer.

Absorption-type refrigerators and freezers

- Check the thermostat.
- Check the heating element.
- If the heating element is working but the refrigerator does not become cool, remove the burner with the tank, or disconnect the refrigerator from the mains. Place upside down for 12 hours, then upright for another 12 hours and re-start normal operation (if the refrigerator or freezer had been transported incorrectly or tilted this action will ensure that the ammonia refrigerant flows back into the correct pipes). If this procedure does not work, send for a qualified refrigeration engineer.

Changing the heating element

1. Disconnect the refrigerator from the mains.
2. Remove the heating element from the chimney.
3. Disconnect from the thermostat.
4. Connect the new element at the ceramic connector or thermostat, using the same terminals.

5. Insert the element into the chimney aperture, making sure it is not placed beside the aperture.

Note: For security reasons, the refrigerant liquid circuit is sealed by the refrigerator manufacturer. It should never be opened, because of the hazardous nature of the liquid.

Spares

Bulb
Heating elements
Thermostats
Wicks
Burner glasses

Tools

Vacuum cleaner or brush
Thermometer

Water purification systems

Pure water is essential for many processes in laboratories and other hospital service departments. The necessary level of purity will depend upon the application for which the water is required. Water purification is expensive; indeed, in the preparation of laboratory chemical reagents, the water may be the most expensive component. Before purchasing and installing a water purification unit, it is, therefore, necessary to define the level of purity required, to avoid excessive and unnecessary expense in producing water that is too pure. Similarly, it is wasteful to use very pure water needed for one task, in another application where such pure water is not required.

The cost of producing water to the required standard of purity will depend upon the purity of the starting material, i.e., the tapwater. This may vary enormously as regards both organic and inorganic content.

There are two main techniques of water purification: demineralization and distillation.

Demineralization

Demineralization systems are particularly suitable for the removal of inorganic ions from water by the use of ion-absorbing resins. They can be easily operated and require no energy input, but they do not remove organic impurities, do not produce sterile water, and may be subject to bacterial contamination, particularly in a warm environment.

Demineralizers contain an insoluble cation exchange resin and an anion exchange resin. These resins may be kept in separate columns (Fig. 2.29) or in a mixed-bed column.

To obtain demineralized water, tapwater is passed through the resin columns, which exchange the solute electrolytes against H^+ and OH^- ions. The conductivity of the deionized water can be measured with a conductivity meter fitted to the outlet of the system.

Fig. 2.29. Ion exchanger.

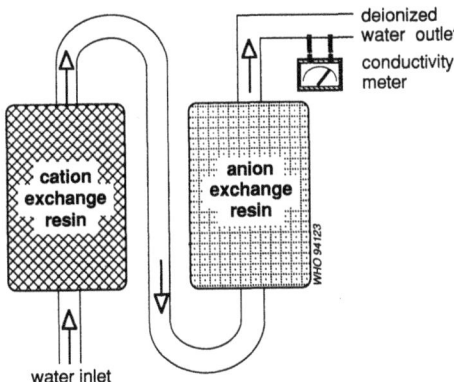

In terms of ion concentration, the water is suitable for most purposes in the laboratory or hospital when the conductivity meter shows less than 20 µS/m. The resins should be regenerated according to the manufacturer's recommendations (or replaced) when the conductivity of the outlet water is greater than 20 µS/m.

The cation exchange resins can be regenerated with hydrochloric acid (HCl), the anion resins with sodium hydroxide solution (NaOH). The intervals between regeneration depend on the quantity of water treated and its hardness. The hardness is related to the calcium content in the water, and may be expressed in mmol/l, or in French or German degrees (°F or °dH). Hardness may be measured chemically by titration with a soap solution.

1 mmol/litre = 9.6 °F or 5.4 °dH

It should be borne in mind that water with a hardness below 0.8 mmol/litre is corrosive, and that the hardness of water treated by a demineralizer is about zero. Thus, demineralized water would need to be mixed with harder water if it were to be fed to a steam boiler, for example, and the piping system would need to be made of a non-corroding material.

Advantages

- The system is easy to operate.
- No energy input is required.
- A supply of pure water is produced immediately.

Demineralization is particularly suited for water supplies with a high content of inorganic ions.

Disadvantages

- In mixed-bed systems, operation depends on a reliable supply of ion-exchange cartridges, which cannot be regenerated.
- The system is vulnerable to bacterial contamination.
- It does not remove organic impurities.
- It does not produce sterile water.

The following points need to be taken into account in order to maintain a continuous and efficient water supply.

- The need for regeneration of the resin will depend upon the ionic content of the water supply.
- The resin must be checked regularly (daily at least) to ensure that it is not saturated and is still producing water to the required level of purity; this is done by measuring the electrical conductivity of the treated water.
- The system must be checked from time to time to ensure that it is leakproof.

- Demineralizers should have a constant flow of water running through in order to reduce the formation of bacterial and fungal colonies. The use of chlorinated water can "poison" the resin in the deionizer, causing premature failure.

Distillation

In water stills, water is purified by evaporation and condensation of the steam. Distilled water may be produced by simple distillation equipment on a small or large scale, according to the need. A water still has the following essential parts (Fig. 2.30):

— water flask (with water feed),
— heating device,
— water condenser system,
— collector.

Fig. 2.30. Laboratory water still.

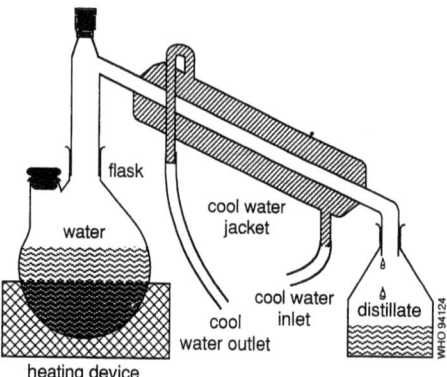

The still may be made of glass, copper, or stainless steel. More sophisticated stills are designed to distil water twice (or more) to obtain a distillate of higher purity. Industrial water stills are constructed differently and can produce several hundred litres of distilled water per day.

Water stills remove organic as well as inorganic material. However, they do not necessarily produce sterile water since spores can be carried over at 100 °C. They are costly to maintain, require water for cooling and a reliable energy source, and should not be used to distil water with a high salt content.

There are a number of safety aspects that need to be considered to ensure the continuous, safe production of pure water:

- A suitable electricity supply (or other energy source), compatible with the equipment's requirements, must be available.
- Constant supervision is required to ensure that there is a sufficient supply of cooling water, the boiling flask does not run dry, and the receiver is not overfilled. Some modern equipment is fitted with trip devices that interrupt the electricity if the boiling flask runs dry.
- As there is an inevitable delay before pure water is produced, the equipment must be switched on in advance, anticipating requirements.
- The boiling flask and element (when it is integrated into the flask) must be checked for inorganic deposits, and descaled as appropriate. This must be done frequently in hard-water areas.
- All glassware must be checked for cracks, especially the boiling flask, which represents a potential safety hazard.
- The system must be checked regularly to ensure that it is leakproof.

Advantages

- The system requires little or no support or maintenance by the manufacturer.
- Water stills remove non-volatile organic, and all inorganic, materials.

Disadvantages

- The system requires close supervision, unless it is fitted with automatic safety devices.
- It requires a supply of cool water for the condenser (this may be a problem in some tropical countries).
- It requires a reliable energy source.
- The relatively large volume of boiling water contained in the glass vessel is a safety hazard.
- Distillation may be impractical for water with a high salt concentration, or for water that is very hard. In this case, desalination by ion exchange may be advisable prior to purification by distillation.

Simple water still

In peripheral laboratories, a simple solar-powered water still can easily be constructed in the open by covering a clean plastic container with an angled glass cover. A fairly large surface area is usually necessary. The water in the container is evaporated by the sun, it condenses on the glass cover and drops into a water collector placed at the lower end of the cover. From there, the distilled water drops through an outlet into a glass bottle underneath the collecting device. Depending on the climatic conditions, 2–7 litres of distilled water with a conductivity of 30–60 µS can be produced daily from a solar still with a surface area of 1 m^2 (Fig. 2.31).

Fig. 2.31. Solar water still.

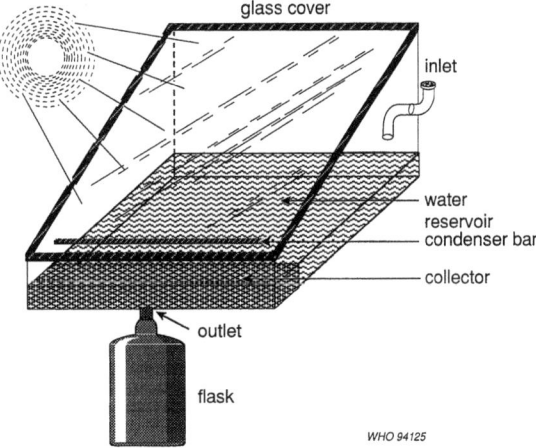

Water filters

Many microorganisms can be removed from water by passing it through a filter of pore size less than 0.75 µm. However, these filters do not remove the smallest microorganisms, such as viruses. The water produced has the same salt concentration as before filtering, and thus if the salt concentration of the available water supply is high, it is preferable to use rainwater when preparing clean water for laboratory investigations.

The following types of filter are used:

- asbestos filters,
- earthenware filters,
- sintered glass filters,
- cellulose membrane filters.

Because of the small pore size of the filters, water passes through slowly. The flow can be accelerated by the application of pressure, or suction of water through the filter.

Storage and handling of deionized and distilled water

Distilled and deionized water can be easily contaminated again by organic materials and microorganisms, which may leach from the container materials into the water. The higher the purity of the water, the more attention must be paid to appropriate storage. Glass or metal containers should not be used for storage of distilled water, since ions, such as silica, magnesium, iron, and lead will leach from the flasks. Clean containers made of polyethylene, polypropylene, or polytetrafluoroethylene are suitable for storage of demineralized and distilled water over long periods.

3. Diagnostic equipment

Some of the equipment described in this and the following sections is used in direct contact with patients and can be hazardous to patients if faulty. Such equipment must, therefore, be used only if it is in full working condition. For this reason, only the simplest maintenance should be carried out by hospital staff without specialized training. For more complex problems, the equipment should be referred to fully trained service personnel, the manufacturer or appointed agents. It is the responsibility of the designated medical, nursing or technical staff who use the equipment to ensure that it is functioning satisfactorily before it is used.

Blood pressure machines (sphygmomanometers)

There are three main types of sphygmomanometer in use:

— mercury type,
— aneroid type,
— electronic type.

The mercury type is preferred since it is the most reliable. Descriptions of the other two types are included here since they are in common use.

Mercury type

This is perhaps the most common type of sphygmomanometer. It consists of a reservoir of mercury, which can be pumped into a manometer tube. This tube lies on a graduated scale which is usually calibrated from 0 to 300 mmHg. The blood-pressure cuff is wrapped round the patient's arm just above the elbow, the machine connected up, and air pumped in using the bulb provided. The cuff is, in turn, connected to the top of the reservoir by a rubber tube. The air pumped into the cuff is under pressure, and this same cuff pressure will be transmitted to the top of the reservoir, pushing the mercury up the calibrated tube. When the pumping of air into the cuff is stopped, the reading on the scale will indicate the pressure in the cuff (Fig. 3.1).

Fig. 3.1. Blood pressure machine—mercury type.

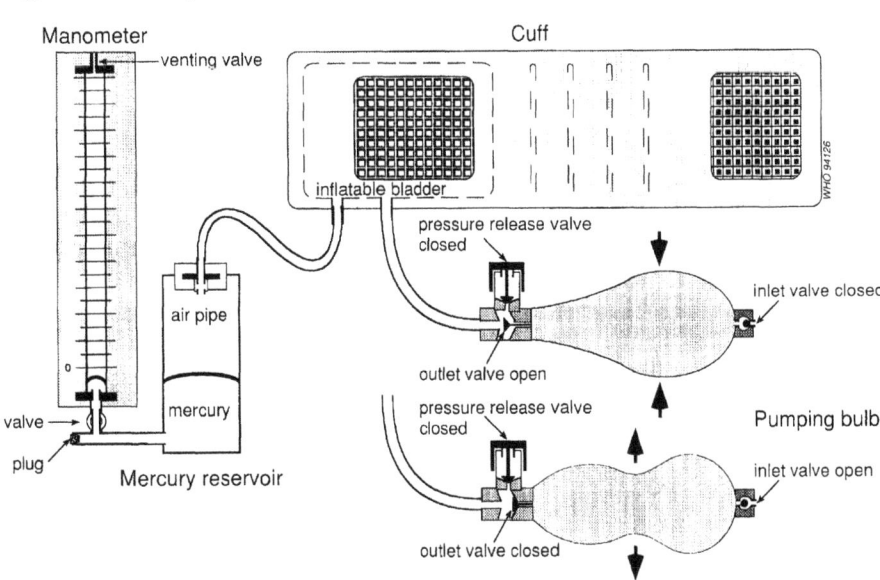

The two non-return valves, the inlet and outlet valves, cause the bulb to act like a pump to create the necessary pressure in the cuff. After the outlet valve, a pressure release mechanism is fitted to permit slow release of the pressure in the cuff when finding the blood pressure.

The cuff is inflated until the pressure as shown on the scale is above the expected blood pressure, and a stethoscope is placed on the artery at the elbow. Because the pressure in the cuff is above the expected blood pressure, no sounds will be heard as the blood cannot flow in the artery that is under the cuff. The cuff pressure is now slowly released by opening the valve on the bulb, the pressure in the cuff falling as the air escapes. At some point, the pressure in the cuff will fall below the blood pressure, blood will start to flow in the artery under the cuff and the sounds of the blood circulation will be heard. As soon as these sounds are heard, the reading on the scale is noted; this is the systolic pressure. As the pressure in the cuff falls further, the sound changes at the point where the cuff pressure equals the diastolic pressure.

It is important that the initial mercury level is adjusted to zero, with no pressure in the cuff. If it is higher, the machine will give falsely high readings; if it is less than zero, it will give falsely low readings. Adjust the level of mercury by undoing the reservoir cap, and with a syringe and needle, add or remove mercury until the level is correct.

The mercury should be clean. With time it tends to become oxidized to mercuric oxide, a black powder. When this happens, remove the mercury and clean the system. Aspirate the dirty mercury into a clean syringe, then filter it through a filter-paper, into a clean receiver. Do this several times until the mercury is clean. Replace the clean mercury and top it up to the zero mark with fresh mercury. Finally, replace the reservoir cap.

Do not handle the mercury more than is necessary, and do not inhale the dust; mercury is a cumulative poison and should be handled with care. Store old mercury in a strong glass jar with a little water floating on the top to stop it fuming. When cleaning the tube and reservoir, blow the dust out with an air-line. Do this outside so that the workplace does not become contaminated.

There is a leather seal at the top of the tube to keep the mercury in. This seal is very important. If it is faulty, the machine may give readings that are too high. This is because, as the mercury falls in the tube, air passes in through the washer at the top. If the air cannot enter the tube quickly enough, the mercury is held back slightly as it falls. This means that the pressure in the cuff will be slightly lower than the reading showing on the scale.

This may be checked as follows:

Pump air into the cuff in the normal way, causing the mercury to rise in the tube. When the inflation stops the mercury should stop rising in the tube. If the washer is faulty, the mercury will continue to rise for a short time, as the air above the mercury continues to pass out of the tube, past the washer. The same phenomenon will occur, in reverse, when the mercury is going in the other direction. The problem can be confirmed by taking the washer out, and repeating the test. The mercury should come to a sudden stop the moment the pumping is stopped. Take care not to pump the mercury too far up the tube, as it will "fountain" out of the top.

The solution to the problem is to change the washer. This may have to be done several times before a suitable one is found. If a satisfactory washer is not available, it is possible to make one out of suitable material, as long as it allows the air to pass at the correct rate, but prevents the mercury from spilling out.

Aneroid type

As the name implies, aneroid sphygmomanometers do not contain any liquid. They are used in the same way as the mercury type, but instead of having mercury in a tube they have a small brass bellows. This is a flat corrugated container into which the air can pass, so keeping it at the same pressure as the cuff. As the pressure inside increases, so the bellows expands, moving a pointer by means of a series of levers and a rack and pinion arrangement. A coiled return spring brings the pointer back to zero when the pressure is released.

This type of machine is much more likely than the mercury type to become damaged and consequently inaccurate. Its accuracy should be checked every 6 months against a mercury machine. The pointer should always return to the zero point when there is no pressure in the cuff.

When checked against a mercury machine, there are two common types of error that may occur with aneroid machines: linear error and non-linear error. With a typical linear error, the two sets of readings might be as follows:

Mercury	*Aneroid*
50 mmHg	60 mmHg
70	80
100	110
150	160

The error (10 mmHg) is the same all the way up the scale.

The following is a typical non-linear error:

Mercury	*Aneroid*
30 mmHg	10 mmHg
50	40
70	70
100	110
150	170

In this case the error changes as the pressure changes.

Correcting either type of error can be time-consuming, and should only be attempted if full details are available in the manual supplied by the manufacturer.

Electronic type

The simplest types of electronic sphygmomanometer have the same cuff and inflation bulb as all the others, and a dial similar to that of the aneroid type. The difference is that in the cuff there is a transducer that picks up the sound of blood flow. This is turned into a note that sounds each time the pulse is detected. These machines are fairly reliable but there may be problems with the connections between the transducer and the instrument; as the units are often sealed, access may be difficult.

The simple electronic machine has no great advantages over the mercury type, and in the long run is likely to be more troublesome. There are more sophisticated types that automatically inflate the cuff at set intervals and give the blood pressure on a digital display. This type of machine does not have a transducer in the cuff, but a very sensitive detector in the body of the machine detects the pulsations in the cuff. The only parts of this machine that can be serviced are the air pump that inflates the cuff, the tubing between the cuff and the pump, and the cuff itself. Most other repairs to these machines would require specialist knowledge.

Ophthalmoscopes and otoscopes

Ophthalmoscope

An ophthalmoscope has two parts:
- the handle, which holds the batteries, the "on/off" switch, and a rheostat that controls brightness;
- the head, which holds the lenses.

Corroded batteries

If the instrument is not in use for any length of time, remove the batteries to prevent corrosion. Removal of batteries that have corroded can be difficult. If the rheostat assembly can be removed from the handle, soaking the handle in boiling water helps to dislodge the batteries. Some handles have a hole in the bottom; in this case introduce a punch through the hole to tap the batteries out. After removal of the batteries, thoroughly clean the handle.

Faulty "on/off" switch or rheostat

First check that the batteries and the bulb are in good condition. With the instrument turned on, check for voltage at the contacts; if there is no voltage, examine the rheostat more closely (and, if possible, remove the rheostat and check for continuity with a meter). Check the continuity of the handle, and also check for corrosion under the spring contact at the bottom of the handle.

The head

This is the most complicated part of the instrument. It contains many small lenses. Light from the bulb passes through a number of lens systems and a small mirror before entering the patient's eye. Some of these systems have their own adjustments, apart from the beam-focusing lenses. Do not attempt to open the head unless you are already experienced in taking the lenses apart and re-assembling them. If the lenses need to be cleaned, try blowing them free of dust with a powerful blower; such a blower can be made from a sphygmomanometer inflation bulb with a blunted needle on the end. If the lenses are very dirty, clean them with methanol and a piece of soft cloth.

Otoscope

The handle of an otoscope is often the same as that of an ophthalmoscope.

The head

The main part of the head holds the bulb, and may also have a lens. On the front, one of a number of different sizes of speculum can be fitted. A set of five specula is normally supplied with the instrument. On the side, there may be a small tubing connector, which is used for inflation. It is important that the head is airtight. Check this by assembling the instrument complete with the tubing connector and inflation bulb (e.g., from a blood pressure machine). With a finger over the end of the speculum, gently squeeze the bulb. There should be no obvious leaks. If there are, check as follows:

- Check that the speculum fits properly and that it is not cracked.
- Check that the tubing nipple is screwed in properly.
- Check that the rear lens fits properly; it may be that the lens is cracked or missing. If so, replacement will be necessary. If a spare lens is not available, use a thin piece of glass; shape it on a slow, water-lubricated grindstone to fit, and then glue it into place. Although the lens effect will be lost, the instrument will still be usable. Do not shape the glass on a high-speed grinder, because it may crack.

If there is no light:

- Check the bulb.
- Check the batteries and the handle as described for ophthalmoscopes.
- Check, with a meter, for continuity between the battery contact and the bulb contact. Use a needle connected to the meter probe to make contact with the bulb contact.

Laryngoscopes

A laryngoscope (Fig. 3.2) is used to examine the pharynx and larynx, and aids the passing of an endotracheal tube into the trachea. It consists of a handle which contains the batteries, and a blade which has a light bulb. The bulb lights up when the blade is opened up and locked into position for use. The blades are available in different shapes and sizes to suit different needs, e.g., for use on adults or children. The most common problem is that the bulb fails to light or just flickers. To determine the cause of the problem:

- Check that the bulb is screwed in tightly, and that it is a good one.
- Check that the batteries have power and that the contacts are clean.

Fig. 3.2. Laryngoscope.

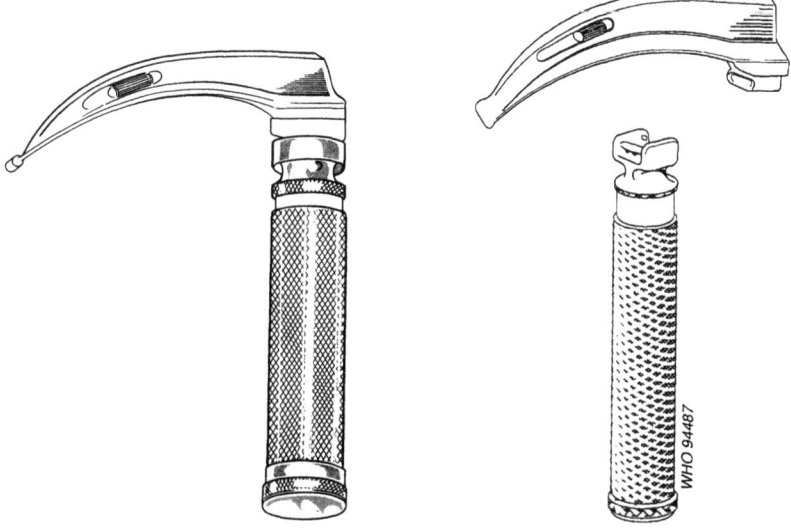

- Clean dirty contacts with sandpaper. The spring at the bottom of the handle often becomes corroded; this may be the cause of the bulb not lighting.

If the laryngoscope still does not work, inspect the contact between the blade and the handle. There is a lead contact, or a stainless steel pin, on the blade, and a brass spring contact pin in the handle. Long use can wear away the lead contacts; if this is the fault, take a soldering iron and reform the lump into a round shape. If the instrument still does not function, check the brass pin. Ensure that it moves in and out correctly, and that it is clean both inside and outside the handle. Install good batteries in the handle, replace the bottom, and check with a meter that there is a voltage at the pin contact.

If the pin is faulty, unscrew the contact and its insulating sleeve with a long, flat-bladed screwdriver. The sleeve may be made of nylon or tufnol (which looks like wood, but is, in fact, cloth and resin). Repair the damaged contact as required. If the laryngoscope still does not function, check (using a multimeter) the continuity between the contact pin at the end of the blade and the body of the blade. This checks the bulb, the contact pin, and the wire between them. If there is no reading, the problem must lie with the wire, the bulb contact, or the connection of the wire to the contact at the base of the blade. Check the wire by clipping one multimeter probe to a fine piece of wire or a needle, and the other probe to the contact at the end of the blade. Carefully introduce the needle into the bulb screw hole so that it touches the bulb contact and not the blade, and check continuity. If there is no continuity there is a problem with the wire. It is possible that it is broken or has become unsoldered. It may be that the contact that touches the bulb has moved too far back into the holder and is not touching the bulb. In either case, it will be necessary to remove the contact and wire and adjust or replace as appropriate.

Proceed as follows:

1. Unsolder the wire at the lead lump end, or pull out the steel pin.
2. Grasp the contact that the bulb touches, and pull the wire through and out of the blade. Take care not to lose the spring and insulating tube behind the bulb contact.
3. Unscrew the lead contact, which is in an insulating threaded insert (made of nylon or tufnol). Telephone wire may be used for rewiring.
4. Unsolder the bulb contact from the faulty piece of wire, and solder it on to the new wire, making sure that the wire is long enough to pass back through the blade.
5. Feed the wire through the blade from the bulb end. It has to pass around a sharp bend, which may be difficult.
6. Cut back the insulation to just below where the threaded bush will end when screwed in place.
7. Screw in the threaded bush, with the bare end of wire passing through the hole. (It may be necessary to re-drill this hole.)
8. Re-solder the wire in place, and smooth the end. If it is a pin type, do not solder, but wrap the wire around the pin.

If the batteries have corroded in the handle to such an extent that it is not possible to remove them in the usual way, use the method described for ophthalmoscopes and otoscopes (page 64).

Check the blade for peeling chrome. This can be sharp. Scrape back to the smooth chrome, sand the rough edges to obtain a smooth finish, and polish.

The newer types of laryngoscope use optical fibres in the blade. The bulb is in the handle and the blade has a bundle of optical fibres to transmit the light to the tip. The blades normally give no trouble, but the handle may give rise to the problems described above.

Stethoscopes

Stethoscopes require little maintenance apart from replacement of lost, cracked, or broken parts, such as ear-pieces and diaphragms (Fig. 3.3). On the older types, the tubing may perish and need replacing. While it is possible to buy proper, but expensive, stethoscope tubing, ordinary tubing of a suitable size may be fitted. Most newer stethoscopes have tubing that does not perish, though it can become sticky if certain chemicals come into contact with it.

Fig. 3.3. Three types of stethoscope with details of chest-pieces.

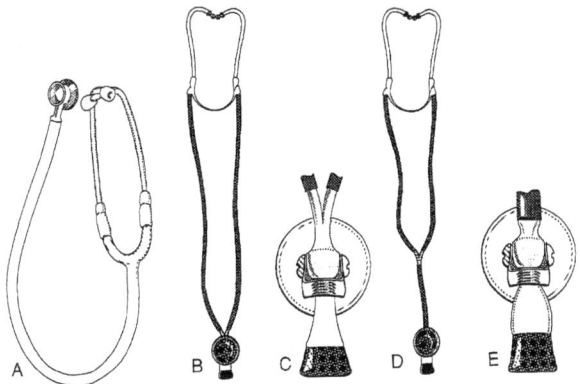

If nothing can be heard through a stethoscope, check whether:

— The earpieces are blocked; if they are, unscrew them, push the blockage out and clean with a little spirit.
— The diaphragm is missing or split; replacements can be purchased or can be made out of a piece of radiographic film or similar plastic sheet.
— The tube is split.

Fetal stethoscopes require no maintenance. The servicing of electronic stethoscopes is outside the scope of this manual.

Electrocardiograph machines and cardiac monitors

Electrocardiograph (ECG) machines are used to monitor the electrical activity of the heart and display it on a small screen or record it on a piece of paper. The electrical activity is picked up by means of electrodes placed on the skin. The signal is amplified, processed if necessary, and then displayed.

There are many types of ECG machine and cardiac monitor, ranging from the very basic, which will just show or write the ECG trace, to complex machines that will give much more information about the status of the heart, and may combine a screen and a paper-writer. These machines run off the mains electricity supply and, in addition, often have internal rechargeable batteries.

Maintenance and safety checking

The following items of test equipment are required:

— a digital multimeter or a good analogue meter;
— a "Megger" (for high-voltage insulation testing);
— a safety checker;
— an ECG simulator (this is an instrument that produces a signal similar to that of the heart and makes workshop testing much easier).

The first two items are essential. A safety checker is not essential, but testing will be limited without it. (If a safety checker is not available, make up an earth-leakage current tester, as described below.) Follow the instructions and the service manual supplied by the manufacturers.

Safety checking is most important. Faulty insulation or earth connections can be serious. Safety checks should be undertaken at least twice a year. Keep a log book with details of each safety check and each reported fault.

The following four tests should be carried out as a minimum (additional tests are possible with a safety checker).

- Earth continuity: using a multimeter, a reading of less than 0.1 ohms should be obtained between the earth pin on the mains plug and the chassis of the unit.
- Mains circuit insulation: using a "Megger", check that there is at least 50 Mohms between the earth pin and live pin, and between the earth pin and the neutral pin, on the mains plug.
- Patient circuit insulation: using a "Megger", check that there is at least 50 Mohms between the patient lead connections and the earth pin and the live pin and the neutral pin on the mains plug. (Conduct the two insulation tests at 500 volts.)
- Earth leakage: using the test equipment illustrated in Fig. 3.4, check that the leakage current is less than 500 microamps.

After safety checking, carefully clean the machine both inside and outside.

Earth-leakage current tester

The 1 kohm resistor should be of a non-inductive type, i.e., a carbon-film resistor, and not wire-wound. Mount the circuit shown in Fig. 3.4 in a box. One side of the box should be fitted with a mains plug. The other side should be wired to a socket into which the appliance to be tested may be plugged. The two test points are mounted on the same face of the box as the socket, but clear of it. Connect the instrument to the mains supply, and plug the equipment under test into the socket of the instrument, then switch on the power.

Fig. 3.4. Earth-leakage current tester.

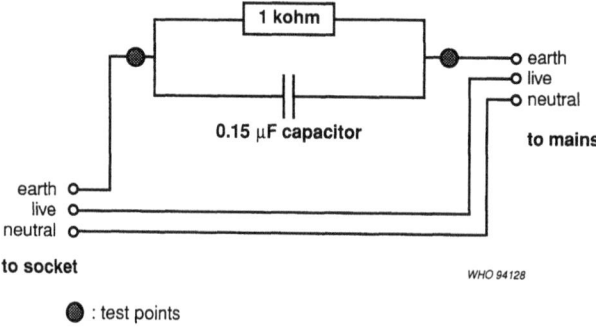

This test equipment is used with a multimeter. Select the AC millivolts setting on the meter and connect it to the points shown. The millivolts reading during the test will be equivalent to microamps. Thus, it should read less than 500 millivolts.

Important spares

Patient electrodes
Patient leads
Styli
Paper

Common faults

When an ECG machine does not work check the following points before taking off the covers to look for electrical/electronic problems:

- Check that the machine is correctly connected to the patient.
- Check that the patient electrode connections are clean and in good condition; dirty or corroded connections will give problems.
- Check that the leads to the patient are in good condition, that the conductor is not broken, and that there is not a short circuit to the cable screening.
- If the machine is being run off its battery, check that the battery is in good condition and that the charger is working correctly.
- Check that the stylus of the writer is heating correctly, and is not worn or damaged.
- Check that there is no mechanical damage, e.g., a broken on/off switch.

If there is no fault with any of these, it is likely that there is an electrical/electronic problem. Send the machine to the manufacturer or appointed agent.

4. Anaesthetic and resuscitation equipment

Breathing machines

Oxford bellows

This is a hand-operated bellows unit for inflating the lungs (Fig. 4.1). It consists of an inlet connection and valve, the bellows in the middle, an outlet valve with outlet connection, and tap. There is a magnet in a holder under the bellows, which is used to immobilize the disk valve when a non-return valve (such as the Ambu) is in use.

Fig. 4.1. Oxford inflating bellows.

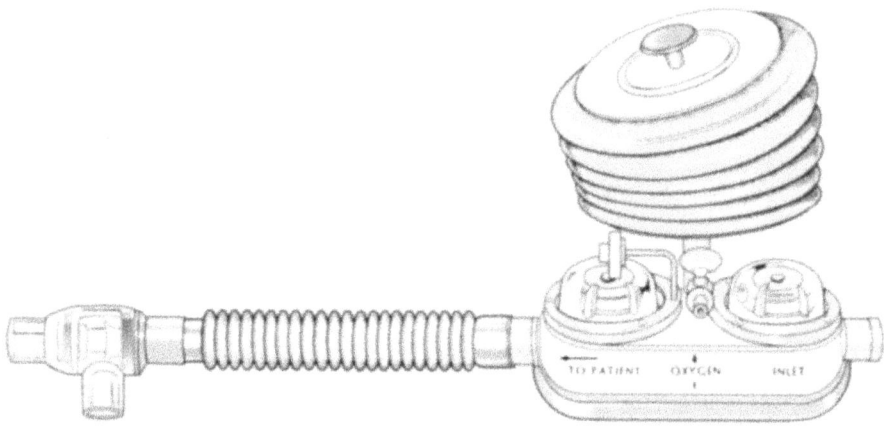

Compression of the bellows, during artificial respiration, will produce a full deflection of the flap valve during inspiration. In order to allow the patient to expire to the atmosphere, a small amount of air must pass back up the corrugated tube towards the bellows to reseat the flap valve. If the outlet flap valve of the bellows unit is not immobilized, air will be unable to pass back and the non-return valve will stick in the inspiration position. The magnet referred to above must therefore be fitted, if a non-return valve is being used.

The adult bellows can be exchanged for a paediatric type by unscrewing it from the base. The paediatric bellows has a full-stroke capacity of about 400 ml, making it easier to ventilate children.

The bellows should be inspected regularly. Possible faults in the bellows are listed below.

- *Cracks in the bellows*

Change the whole unit or just the bellows, as appropriate. To replace the bellows, proceed as follows:

1. Remove the bottom plate first, by taking out the four small screws, and then levering off the plate, which is cemented in place with an adhesive.
2. Loosen the inner bottom plate.
3. Access can then be gained to the ball-ended bolt that is attached to the top plate.

4. Holding the bolt with a pair of pliers or spanner, unscrew the knob on top of the bellows, releasing the bolt, spring, and bottom plate. The old bellows can then be pulled off the top plate.
5. Remove all the old cement from the end-plates.
6. Insert the inner top plate into the bellows, apply a small but continuous ring of glue to the groove in the outer top plate, position this on the bellows, and insert the knob.
7. Insert the spring into the bellows from the outer end, apply the ball-ended bolt, and tighten the knob.
8. Glue can then be applied to this thread to seal it. Care must be taken to keep the bellows and the plates concentric during tightening.
9. Stretch the bellows over the inner bottom plate and position the ring on the bellows' edge, in the groove in the plate.
10. Apply glue to the groove in the outer bottom plate and to the threads of the four small screws.
11. Assemble the bottom plate with the screws, again ensuring concentricity of the rubber in the grooved end-plate.
12. Allow the glue to dry for at least 1 hour before testing the bellows for leaks.

- *Cracks in the glass domes*

Replace the glass dome. (Note that the metal clamping rings are not interchangeable between the inlet and outlet valves.) It is advisable to use new gaskets with new glasses, and to tighten the fixing screws in rotation, a little at a time, so as not to stress the glass unevenly. Always ensure that the magnetic disc valve is installed in the outlet valve assembly, after dismantling the valve body.

- *Inoperative magnet*

If the magnet fails to lift the outer valve clear of the valve seating, check that the magnet is functioning, that the disc is the correct one, and that it is magnetic.

- *Faulty outlet valve*

Check the outlet valve by first replacing the magnet in its storage holder; block the inlet port with a cork, and attempt to extend the bellows. It should not be possible to extend the bellows more than 2.5 cm in 1 minute.

- *Leaks in the inlet valve*

To check the inlet valve, block the outlet port with a cork and attempt to compress the bellows. Again, movement should not exceed 2.5 cm in 1 minute. Remove the cork.

Penlon bellows unit

This is similar to, but simpler than, the Oxford bellows unit. It has a single flap and was designed specifically for use with a non-return valve. It must **never** be used with a simple spring-loaded expiratory valve. The maintenance of these units is similar to that for the Oxford bellows. The commonest site for leaks is at the base of the concertina bellows, where it is connected to the valve unit with a nut and washer. Both bellows are capable of delivering a volume of about 1300 ml; a 10-cm stroke will deliver about 800 ml.

Infant incubators

Infant incubators (Fig. 4.2) are used to keep unwell newborn or premature infants in controlled conditions of temperature, humidity, and oxygen level. Doors are provided in the sides to allow access to attend to the infant. The common types incorporate a low-power heater and a fan to circulate the air. There are warning alarms to draw attention to mains failure or overheating, for example.

Fig. 4.2. Infant incubator.

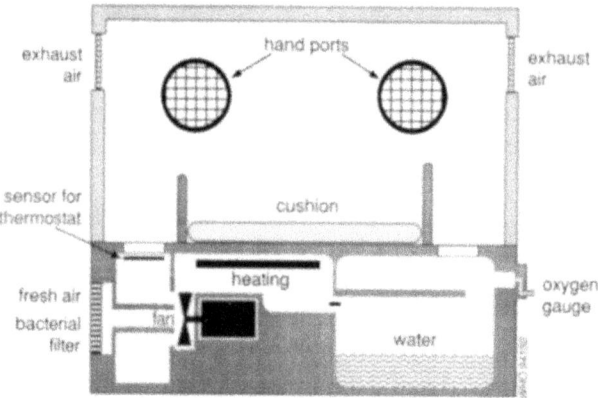

Maintenance

Day-to-day care involves care of the door catches and seals. Like ventilators and anaesthetic machines, the incubator needs to be thoroughly checked twice a year, and functioning should be checked after each cleaning. Check that:

- it warms up to, and is able to maintain, the set temperature;
- the over-temperature alarm works at the correct setting;
- all dials read correctly.

Also check the electrical safety of the machine. Problems are most likely to be of an electrical nature. If there is overheating, check that the ambient air temperature is not too high, and that the machine is not exposed to the sun. A fan-failure alarm may indicate that the bearings of the fan motor need lubricating or replacing. Correct bearings may be available from a supplier of roller bearings for industrial use.

Do not attempt to repaint the interior surfaces. This can cause serious harm to newborn infants by contaminating the air they breathe. Special repainting procedures are available from manufacturers, upon request.

General cleaning

Cleaning may be carried out with soap and clean water. All the surfaces and corners should be washed and dried thoroughly, using plenty of clean absorbent paper, or clean cloth, to ensure that every corner is completely dry. Any remaining moisture can promote the growth of bacteria. If the canopy is made of Perspex, clean it with soap and water, but do not use abrasive compounds. Finally, wipe the canopy with a little ethanol (70%).

Full disinfection

1. Remove any porous material from the incubator.
2. Place a bowl of formaldehyde solution (formalin) in the incubator (about 250 ml).

3. Turn on the incubator, and leave it to heat with the fan circulating the air, for at least 1.5 hours.
4. Remove the bowl of formaldehyde solution, and replace it with a bowl of 200 g/l ammonia solution. Leave for 1.5 hours with the fan and heating switched on. The ammonia removes the smell of the formalin.
5. Remove the ammonia solution, strip the machine down and clean with soap and water. If after cleaning there is still some residual smell of formalin, leave the incubator running until all the smell has disappeared.

Notes on formaldehyde

A stock solution of formaldehyde in water (370 g/l), generally called formalin, should be available. Prior to disinfection, the equipment should be cleaned of all gross contamination and then arranged to permit a free flow of formaldehyde vapour over all potentially infected surfaces. The properties of formaldehyde make it unsuitable for the disinfection of porous substances such as filters and fabrics, including all bedding material. Any such material should be removed and cleaned by other means. The disinfecting process should take place at a temperature above 20 °C.

Methanol is often added to formalin as a stabilizer if it is to be stored for long periods. Methanol prevents polymerization. When buying formalin for disinfection, do not select an industrial grade as this may well have up to 10% methanol added. Such a high concentration of methanol can damage some plastics, including Perspex. Buy formalin containing not more than 1% methanol. Always store formalin in a dark-coloured bottle, out of the sunlight.

Oxygen entrainment systems

An entrainer is used to administer an air/oxygen mixture to patients. Fig. 4.3 shows how an entrainer works.

Oxygen from a flowmeter enters the entrainer and draws in air via the air entrainment duct. The duct is covered by a regulator disc, which can be rotated and has holes in it of different sizes. As the disc is turned, different size holes can be lined up with the entrainment duct. In the diagram, the disc has been turned so that the largest hole, marked 40, is against the orifice. At this setting, the flow of oxygen pulls in 3 times its own volume of air, so the mixture administered to the patient is 40% oxygen (because the air also contains some oxygen). The disc can

Fig. 4.3. How an entrainer works.

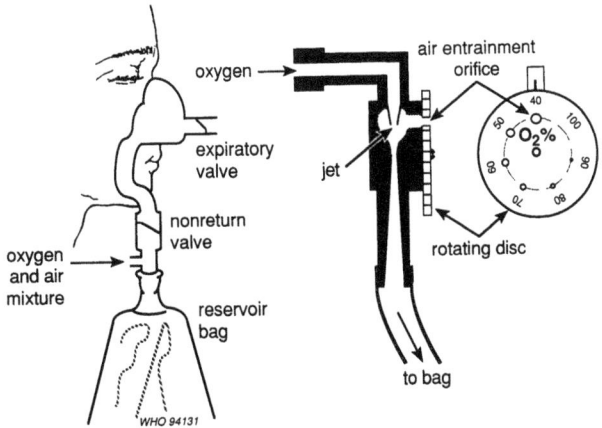

be rotated to a smaller hole, resulting in a higher oxygen concentration being delivered to the patient because less air is taken in. If the disc is turned to 100, the patient will receive 100% oxygen, as there is no inlet for air. Once the disc has been set, the patient will receive a gas mixture with the same proportion of oxygen, whatever the flow rate.

The maintenance of such a basic entrainer is simple, and consists of making sure that the holes in the disc and the jet are not blocked, and that the disc is free to be rotated, though not so free that it can be turned by accident. When checking or unblocking the holes or jet, do not use a drill or wire, as this may alter the size of the hole and thus the amount and composition of gas that is delivered to the patient.

Farman entrainer

This is an entrainer designed for paediatric use (Fig. 4.4). It can be used with an Epstein-Macintosh-Oxford (EMO) machine to vaporize ether, or with an Oxford Miniature Vaporizer (OMV) to vaporize other anaesthetic agents. The entrainer consists of a fine jet through which oxygen passes into a venturi-shaped tube, drawing in air.

Fig. 4.4. Farman entrainer.

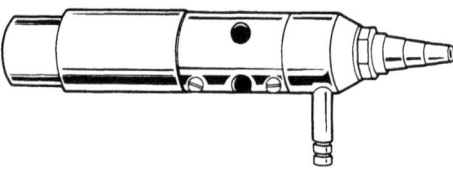

The entrainer is plugged into the inlet of an EMO machine and a blood pressure gauge attached to the side-arm. Oxygen from a cylinder is passed through the entrainer, the flow being adjusted until the blood pressure gauge reads 100 mmHg. At this setting, the entrainer will deliver a flow of 10 litres of oxygen-enriched air per minute; the gas mixture will contain about 35% oxygen.

Remember, ether and oxygen mixed in air form an explosive mixture. When testing an entrainer, it is safer to fix it to an empty EMO or carry out the test in a well-ventilated area.

If the outflow of the entrainer is blocked, the high-pressure gas will escape from the air-inlet ports and the maximum pressure in the system will be about 11 mmHg (15 cm H_2O or equivalent on the gauge in use). Thus, if for any reason the gases are prevented from escaping from the breathing circuit, the maximum pressure of gas the patient will receive is about 11 mmHg. A fine filter is provided at the air-inlet port to prevent dust from entering the high-pressure chamber and damaging the jet. Do not clean the jet by probing it with a piece of wire, as this may alter the size of the jet. There is also a wire gauze to protect the air entry port. Make sure the filters are clear and check the jet, which may be removed for cleaning. This entrainer is cheap to buy, economical, safe, and simple in construction; it is easy to maintain (as outlined above) and, if treated with care, will last a long time.

Systems for continuous-flow anaesthesia

Continuous-flow anaesthetic machines (commonly known as Boyle's machines or simply gas machines) are in widespread use. They rely on a supply of compressed medical gas, either from cylinders attached directly to the machine or piped from a large bank of cylinders or liquid oxygen supply elsewhere in the hospital. The two gases most commonly used are oxygen and nitrous oxide. Cylinders are attached to the machine by a special yoke that prevents the connection of the nitrous oxide supply to the oxygen port and vice versa – the pin-index system. Some older machines may lack this system, and extreme care is needed in their use to prevent incorrect connections. The cylinders contain gas at high pressure, which is reduced to the anaesthetic machine's working pressure, usually 400 kPa (4 atmospheres), by a reducing valve. Each gas then passes through a needle valve at the base of a rotameter. This valve controls the flow of gas to the patient, once the cylinder valve has been opened with a key or spanner to allow gas to flow out. The gas passes through the rotameter, which measures the gas flow by upward displacement of a bobbin in a tube, and along the "back bar" at the top of the machine, where it may be diverted through a vaporizer for the addition of a volatile anaesthetic agent (Fig. 4.5). A separate switch or tap is usually provided to allow for a high flow of oxygen to be delivered to the patient in case of emergency, bypassing the rotameters and vaporizers. Gas is delivered from the common gas outlet at the top or front of the machine, to which a breathing system is connected.

Fig. 4.5. Gas pathway on a continuous-flow (Boyle's) machine with a compressed gas supply: (1) pressure gauges, (2) reducing valves, (3) flow-control (needle) valves, (4) rotameters, (5) calibrated vaporizer, (6) Boyle's bottle, (7) Magill breathing system.

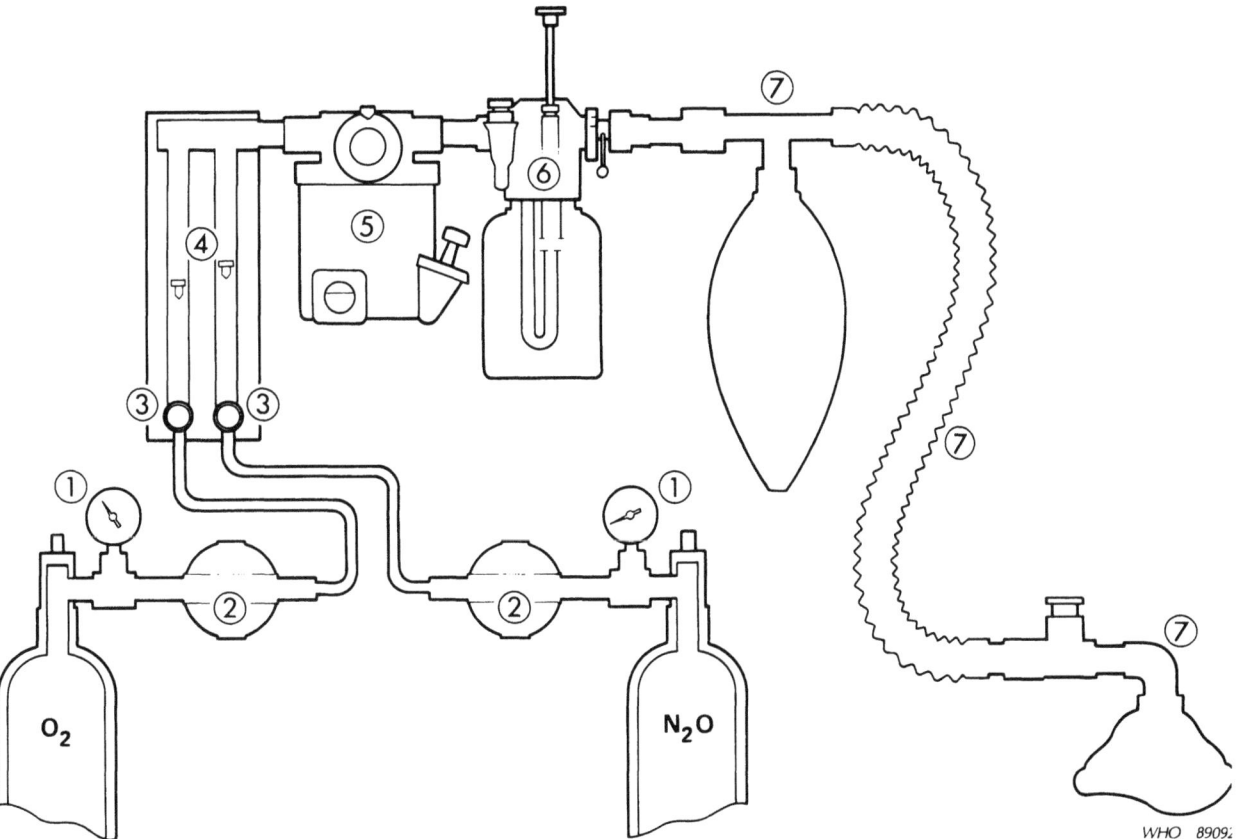

Flowmeter unit

The servicing of a flowmeter, as for example the one shown in Fig. 4.6, is carried out as described below.

Fig. 4.6. Flowmeter.

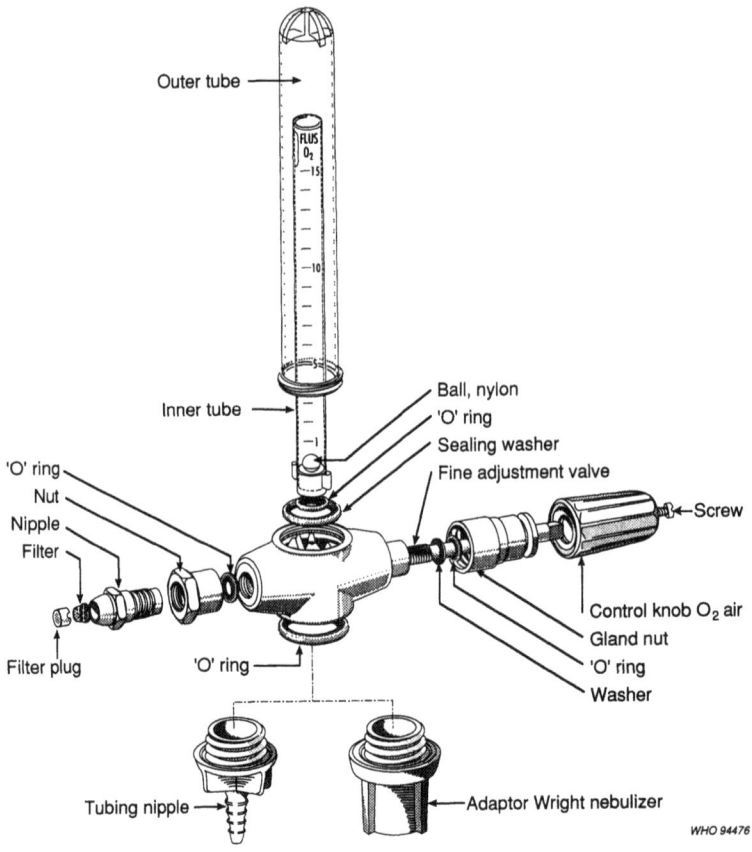

1. Disconnect the flowmeter from the gas supply and remove the tubing nipple or nebulizer from the outlet of the flowmeter. Inspect the tubing nipple O-ring for damage and replace, as necessary.
2. Hold the flowmeter vertically, unscrew and remove the outer tube and inspect it for dirt and damage. Clean or replace it, as necessary.
3. Remove the inner tube, spider (not illustrated), and nylon ball. Inspect all three parts for dirt and damage, and clean or replace, as required.
4. Examine the O-ring and seal in the body of the unit, and replace them if damaged. Lightly grease with silicone grease. Remove excess grease. Examine the threads in the body of the flowmeter. If they are damaged, do not attempt to repair them, but replace the body.
5. Check the fine-adjustment control valve for smooth operation. If the valve is not smooth through its whole range of movement, proceed as follows:

   - *Ensure that the valve is closed.* Remove the label from the end of the control knob, and check the knob for cracks. Replace if necessary.
   - Remove the screw that holds the control knob to the valve spindle and pull the knob off, then look inside for cracks. Replace the knob if there are any.
   - Unscrew the gland nut and inspect the thread for damage. Replace if there is any. Clean if required.
   - Examine the gland nut packing bush for serviceability, and replace if necessary. For replacement, lightly grease the spindle and bush, and then remove the excess grease.
   - Unscrew and withdraw the valve assembly. Examine the O-ring and seal for serviceability, and replace as necessary. If they are replaced, lightly grease the O-ring and seal, and remove the excess grease.
   - Examine the valve threads for damage, and replace the valve assembly, if necessary.

- Fit the O-ring and seal into the flowmeter body and screw the valve assembly home. Tighten to the torque recommended in the manufacturer's service book.
- Fit the gland nut and tighten sufficiently to maintain a gas-tight seal, but not so tight as to restrict the smooth operation of the fine-adjustment control valve.
- Replace the control knob and secure it to the valve spindle with the screw.

6. Check the inlet adaptor assembly for security of attachment and damage. Replace if damaged. If it is loose, remove the assembly, coat the threads with a suitable liquid for sealing nuts on threads, and screw home.
7. Remove the filter plug and the filter. Examine the filter for dirt, refit or replace, as necessary, and press home the filter plug.
8. Connect the flowmeter to a 300–400 kPa, 300–400 litre oxygen supply, and with a leak-test fluid, such as soapy water, carry out a leak test with the flowmeter pressurized. There should be no leaks. Finally clean the flowmeter.

After-service testing

When servicing and any repairs have been completed, carry out the following tests:

- Connect a gas supply of 400 kPa to the inlet of the flowmeter. Connect a suitable length of tubing to the tubing nipple at the flowmeter outlet, and attach the other end of the tube to an accurate flowmeter. Carry out the checks listed below.
- Check that the two flowmeters agree at the following settings:

    2.0 (± 0.5) litres per minute
    5.0 (± 0.5) litres per minute
    10.0 (± 1.0) litres per minute
    15.0 (± 1.0) litres per minute

    All readings must be taken at the centre of the ball.
- Check that each setting is easily obtained and steady.
- If the above flow rates cannot be achieved, check all seals and O-rings, and retest. If the required flow rates still cannot be achieved, replace the inner tube or ball. If the flow rates are still not correct, check the fine adjustment valve again.

Remember that the outer tube is at the pressure of the regulator; do not remove it when the system is pressurized.

Faults

- Unable to obtain full flow:
    - Check and clean the fine adjustment valve.
    - Outlet partially blocked: unblock it.
    - Low cylinder pressure: fit a full cylinder.
    - Regulator pressure set very low: adjust to the correct pressure.

- A small flow showing when the fine adjustment valve is turned off:
    - There may be a crack in the flow-tube outer tube.
    - The outer cover may not be screwed on properly.

- Ball bounces with a popping noise:
    - This is called motor-boating, and is caused by a dirty valve seat.

Rotameter tube

Many machines use a tube called a rotameter to measure the gas flow. A true rotameter tube is made of electrically conductive glass, and has a tapered bore, which is wider at the top than at the bottom. Inside, there is a bobbin with flutes cut out at the top, which make the bobbin spin in the gas flow, showing that it is not stuck. The bobbin is usually made of aluminium, which is light and resistant to corrosion. However, some corrosion may still occur, and it is therefore important that, during the servicing, the tube is taken out. Remove the bobbin, and make sure that every part of it is absolutely dry. If the bobbin has started to corrode, this is what to do:

1. Remove the tube very carefully from the block.
2. Remove the bobbin stop, at the top of the tube.
3. If it is free, tip the bobbin out of the tube. If it is not free, place a thin piece of wood, that is just smaller in diameter than the inside of the tube, into the tube and tap the bobbin with it to try and force it out. This must be done with the greatest of care, as excessive force will crack the tube. If in difficulty, try a little penetrating oil.
4. Once the bobbin is out, clean with very fine abrasive paper, removing all signs of corrosion, and leaving the area smooth.
5. Clean the tube of any corroded material, and dry thoroughly.
6. Replace the bobbin in the tube, and replace the tube in the block.
7. Test the assembly to ensure that the bobbin does not stick in the tube.

The graduations on the tube are calibrated with the bobbin inside. The bobbin has a number on it, and the same number should be on the glass tube. The bobbin should not be changed from one tube to another (except in an emergency) as this will make the graduations slightly inaccurate. Tubes cannot be used for different gases either, as each tube is calibrated only for the gas that is marked on it. In any case, the tubes are often of different sizes and physically will not fit into the wrong place. They should have an accuracy of about $\pm 2\%$.

Other flow indicators

Coxeter dry-bobbin flowmeter

A bobbin floats in a vertical glass tube of uniform bore. Gas enters from below. As the flow increases the bobbin rises in the tube and allows the gas to pass out through a series of holes in the back of the tube. This flowmeter has been largely replaced by more accurate types of rotameter.

Bryce-Smith induction unit

This is a simple and reliable addition to the EMO for delivering limited dosages of halothane. The unit has no controls. Halothane is poured into the measuring dish on the top, which has a capacity of about 3 ml. The wick unit is removed from the bottom and placed in the dish. The wick absorbs the halothane and is then replaced on the bottom of the unit, and will immediately deliver the anaesthetic vapour to the patient. The unit, which is normally left attached to the outlet of the EMO, delivers about 2–4% halothane for 3–4 minutes.

The only maintenance that can be undertaken is to ensure that the wick is in good condition, and that the tapers are not damaged where the unit plugs into the EMO.

Vaporizers

Oxford miniature vaporizer (OMV)

This is a small vaporizer (Fig. 4.7) which can be used to administer anaesthetics. It works in the same way as the larger vaporizers, but does not have a built-in temperature compensation device. However, the base is filled with antifreeze to help stabilize the internal temperature. A number of different versions are available, each of which can be fitted with different scales for use with different anaesthetic agents.

Fig. 4.7. Oxford miniature vaporizer: (1) inlet port; (2) outlet port; (4) water jacket; (6) vaporizing chamber; (8) filling port for anaesthetic; (9) anaesthetic-level indicator.

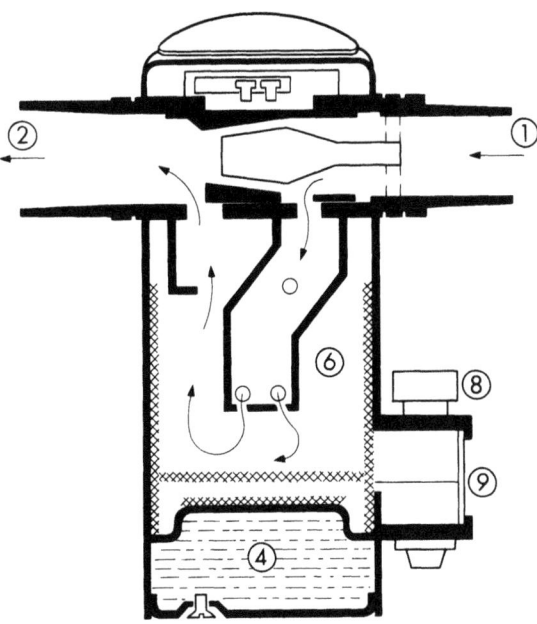

The volatile anaesthetic liquids contain non-volatile substances such as thymol. These accumulate inside the vaporizer and will adversely affect performance, if present in excessive quantities. Removal of the deposits is therefore an essential part of the maintenance of vaporizers. Simple cleaning can be undertaken quite easily and requires no tools. It should be carried out as soon as any stiffness is noticed in the control pointer. However, major cleaning will require special tools and should only be necessary on rare occasions.

Simple cleaning procedure

1. Put a rubber bung into the inlet and turn the vaporizer on to its side, with the outlet port pointing upwards.
2. Pour cleaning fluid (methanol or ether) into the outlet, while moving the pointer to and fro.
3. The vaporizer should be completely filled and allowed to stand for 5 minutes before emptying.
4. The vapour of the cleaning fluid that is left in the vaporizer should be completely removed by opening the control fully and blowing air through the vaporizer for 15–20 minutes with an inflating bellows.

Major cleaning procedure

If possible, refer to the manufacturer's service manual.

1. Remove the pointer by removing the screw and the washer. Lift off the pointer and abutment washer, and remove the scale (Fig. 4.8).

Fig. 4.8. Detail of the Oxford miniature vaporizer.

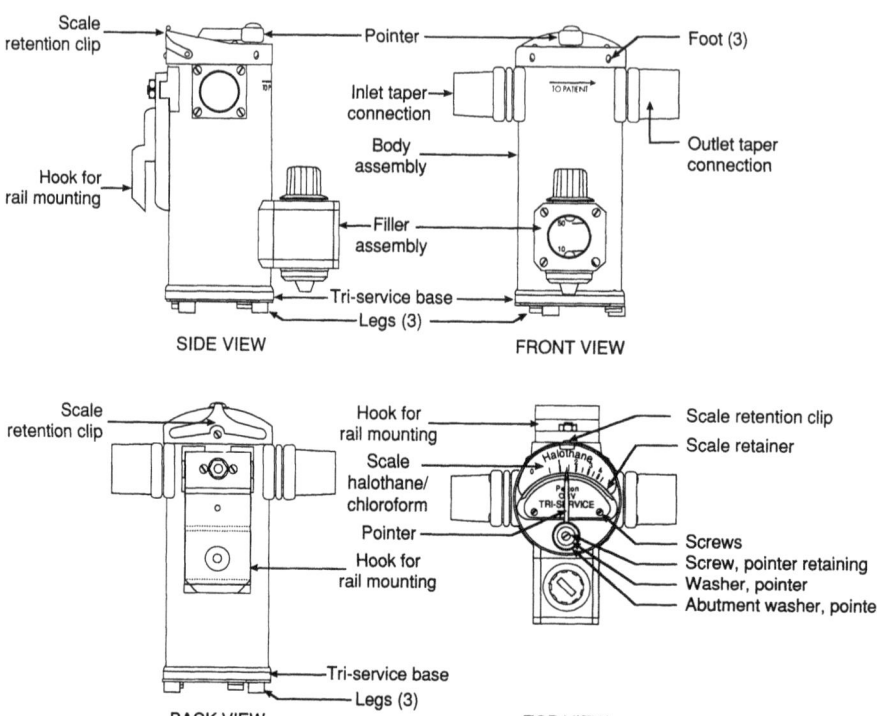

2. Take out the three screws from the lid, and lever the lid off the body. **Note**: These screws are rather short and have a fine thread; treat them very carefully, otherwise the thread will be stripped on the screw or on the vaporizer. Should this happen, it will have to be re-tapped, and a bigger screw fitted.
3. Remove the M6 nut and washer, and take off the "off-line" hook (Fig. 4.9). Remove the two screws, and take off the tenon block and clamp.

Fig. 4.9. Detail of the Oxford miniature vaporizer: top view (pointer and scale removed).

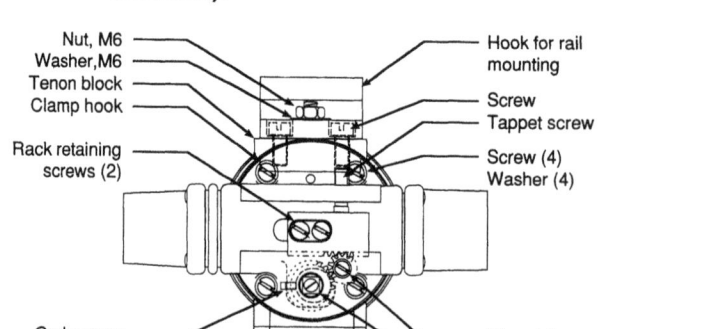

4. Remove the four screws and washers. Lift out the regulator assembly, O-seal, and clamp ring.
5. Part-fill the vaporizing chamber with cleaning liquid (as above). Shake gently to wet all parts of the wicks. Allow to soak for 2–3 minutes and shake it again; repeat this several times. Discard the liquid. Repeat the process until the discarded liquid appears clean. Invert the chamber and allow to dry completely.
6. If the indicator glass is still dirty after the above process, remove the four screws securing it, lift out the glass and wipe clean. Replace the glass, ensuring that the seals and centring ring are replaced in the correct position.
7. If corrosion is present on the wick, e.g., rusty patches, reassemble the vaporizer and return it to the manufacturer for replacement of the wicks.
8. Dismantle the regulator assembly:

   – Remove the inlet and outlet cones (4 screws each), gaskets, and obturator assembly (Fig. 4.10).

Fig. 4.10. Detail of the Oxford miniature vaporizer: cut view, side.

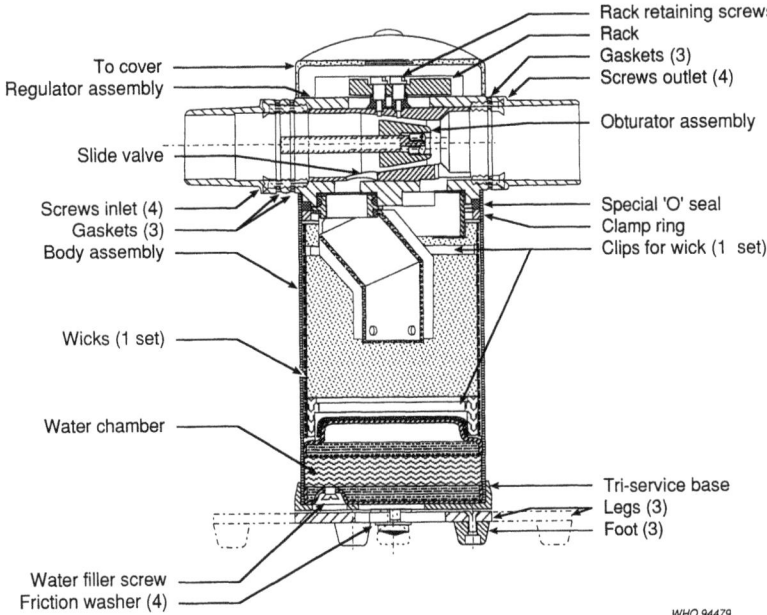

   – Remove the two screws securing the rack. Lift off the rack and spacers. Note that the plastic sleeves inside the spacers must be retained. Also note the relative position of the ports[1] and the direction of the cone of the slider.
   – Remove the slide-valve by pushing from the outlet end of the regulator housing. If it is stiff, use a wooden or plastic drift (stick) to push it out. Do not use metal, as this will damage the machined surfaces.
   – Soaking the assembly in ether or alcohol will usually dissolve the deposits that are causing the stiffness.
   – Wash the slide-valve and regulator housing in cleaning fluid and dry with a clean cloth, paying particular attention to the sliding surfaces. **Never** clean these with abrasive compounds. Metal polish may be used to remove stubborn dirt after first carefully removing the residues and before reassembly.

---

[1] Modern versions have markings on the ports so that they can be realigned in the correct position. Older versions may not have these markings, so, before taking the assembly apart, scratch a line with a screwdriver over the connecting parts.

- Refit slide-valve to housing.
- **Do not** use any oil or grease. Check for smooth motion from one end of the housing to the other.
- Check the location of ports and the direction of the cone, and reassemble the rack with spacers and screws, lining up the marked tooth rack between the two marked teeth on the idler pinion, and, at the same time, the marked teeth on the idler and the pointer pinion.

9. Backlash can develop between the rack and idler, or between the idler and pinion.

    - A tappet screw is provided to adjust the engagement of the former.
    - The pinion is mounted in an eccentric bush, and engagement with the idler is adjusted by slackening the lock screw, rotating the eccentric bush, using a 3-mm bar in the hole provided, until the engagement is correct, and then tightening the lock screw.

10. Reassemble the reducing valve assembly body

    - The special PTFE[1]-coated O-ring that seals the assembly must be examined for damage, and repeated if necessary.
    - Separate the clamp ring and regulator housing by removing the four screws and washers.
    - Insert the clamp ring into the body with the four screw-holes at 45 degrees to the reducing-valve housing, in plan.
    - Immerse the O-ring in warm water (40–50 °C) for a few minutes, to soften it.
    - Place the O-ring on top of the clamp ring.
    - Insert the regulator housing assembly using the 3-mm tommy bar to line up the screw holes in the clamp ring and regulator housing. Insert the draw-screws into two diagonally opposite holes to draw the clamp ring into the body (hand-tight only).
    - Insert two screws and washers, remove draw-screws, and insert the two remaining screws and washers.
    - Tighten all four screws evenly and fully, making sure the regulator is pressed home fully into the body without gaps beneath inlet and outlet square section.

11. Examine the obturator assembly to ensure that the adjustment screws are sealed. If the seal is broken it is advisable to return the unit to the manufacturer. Assemble the gaskets, obturator assembly, and inlet connector with four screws to the reducing-valve housing. Check that the obturator is concentric with the slide-valve. Assemble the gasket and outlet connector to the regulator housing.

12. Test the main body seal for leaks:
    - With the slide-valve open, block the outlet connector and apply pressure to approximately 180 mmHg through the inlet connector.
    - Run a small quantity of cleaning fluid (ether or alcohol) into the joints between the regulator assembly and the body.
    - Check for bubbles.
    - Tighten screws or replace O-ring, if necessary, to obtain a leak-free joint.
    - Tip out any surplus liquid, and allow the machine to dry completely.

13. Reassemble the tenon block, clamp, off-line mounting block, lid, and pointer (reverse of dismantling instructions). Do not fit the scale at this stage.

---

[1] Polytetrafluoroethylene.

Check pointer setting

Do this by inserting a setting gauge, OMV 1, through the outlet side into the valve port, with the pointer between 50 and 60 on the engraved scale on the lid. Move the pointer towards the left until no further movement is possible. The pointer should then indicate 35 on the engraved scale. A positional error of ± 1 mm is acceptable. If the gear train has been wrongly assembled, an error of 7.5 degrees per tooth will be introduced, so that the errors are easy to detect. Remove the setting gauge, assemble the outlet connector and gasket with four screws, and fit the scale back in place.

Testing for leaks

This procedure should be carried out if the unit is reported to be giving low concentrations or is using excessive quantities of halothane or trichloroethylene. Connect the vaporizer to a reservoir, pressure gauge, and air source, as shown in Fig. 4.11. Pump air into the system until a pressure reading of approximately 210 mmHg (28 kPa) is reached. Clamp off the air-supply line with a pair of forceps. The pressure in the system will fall slowly; use a stopwatch to record the time taken for it to fall from 200 mmHg to 190 mmHg.

Fig. 4.11. Leak test layout.

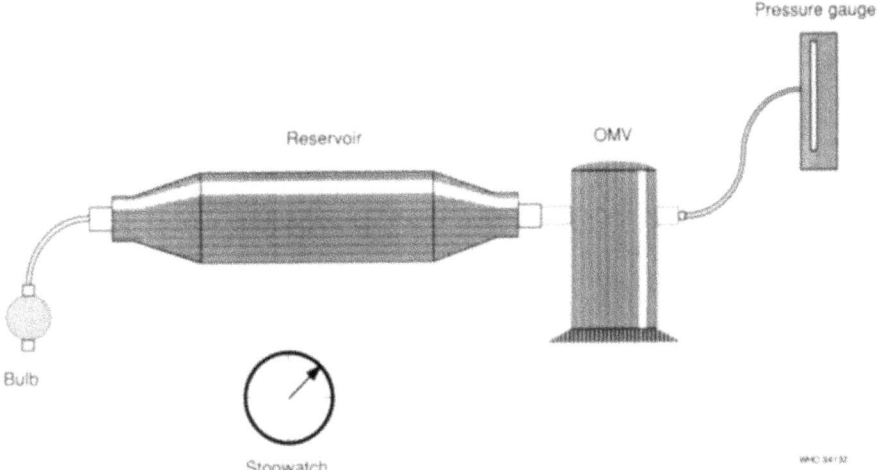

Carry out the test with:

- The control pointer in the OFF position to test the connectors and the top of the regulator housing. Acceptable value: 30 seconds or more.
- The control pointer in the "3.5" position to test the vapour chamber joints. Acceptable value: 30 seconds or more.
- The control pointer in the OFF position and the filler held open to test the vapour seals. Acceptable value: 15 seconds or more.

If the vaporizer does not pass this test, look for the position of the leak by brushing soap solution around the suspect joints while maintaining the internal pressure. Bubbles will form at the leak site. Do not apply soap solution to the opening around the rack, where it could enter the slide valve (once it dries, it will cause the slider to stick).

Note: There is always a certain amount of leakage from the slide-valve but this can be ignored if the test figures above can be obtained.

Specific repairs

Fitting a new level-indicator glass

Remove the four screws, take off the retainer, the old glass, seals, and centring ring. When fitting a new glass, always use new seals. Glasses vary a little in thickness. Three seals are provided in the spare-parts kit, and sufficient seals should be used to obtain good compression on the glass when the retainer is screwed back into place. Test the unit for leaks after fitting a new level-indicator glass.

Fitting a new drain seal

1. Remove the drain screw.
2. Use a pin spanner to unscrew the old drain-seal assembly from the filler block.
3. Discard the old assembly and seal.
4. Fit a new assembly and seal.
5. Tighten securely.
6. Test for leaks.

Fitting a new back seal

1. If a leak develops between the filler block and body, remove the retaining level-indicator glass.
2. With a screwdriver, lever out the engraved back plate of the level indicator; this will expose the heads of two socket-head screws.
3. If tightening does not cure the leak, remove the screws, lift off the filler block and fit a new seal between the block and the body.
4. Reassemble all parts and test for leaks.

Replacing a folding leg (where fitted)

Remove the screw securing the leg to the base, and fit a new leg and new friction washer. The legs are made of malleable material and will withstand flattening with a soft-faced mallet.

To tighten a loose leg (where fitted)

Remove the screw securing the leg to the base, and replace the friction washer. Reassemble.

Replacing the complete base

The complete base assembly, with its feet, is fixed to the body using adhesive. If this joint should be broken as the result of a fall, a suitable adhesive should be used to refix the base. Clean off the old adhesive before refixing, and ensure that the recess in the base is aligned with the water-filling screw.

Other repairs

Faults requiring the instrument to be returned to the manufacturer or agent:

– broken pointer,
– corroded wicks,
– broken seal on obturator.

The vaporizer should be recalibrated every two years by the manufacturer or agent.

Equipment required for servicing

Leak testing

A source of compressed air, at about 200 mmHg (26 kPa). In the absence of a mechanical pump, this may be provided by a blood pressure machine, a hand bulb, or an Oxford inflating bellows.
Rubber bungs to fit the inlet and outlet of the vaporizer, one with a 6-mm tube through it.
A reservoir of capacity 4 litres capable of withstanding a pressure of 200 mmHg (26 kPa).
A pressure gauge to read to 200 mmHg (26 kPa).
Liquid soap solution and a small brush.
Ether or methylated spirit.
A stopwatch.
A pair of clamping forceps.
Rubber or plastic tubing to fit a 6-mm tube.

General servicing equipment (Fig. 4.12)

Setting gauge.
Drain plug key (spanner).
Draw screws.

Fig. 4.12. General servicing equipment.

Setting gauge

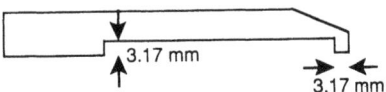

Drain plug key (spanner)

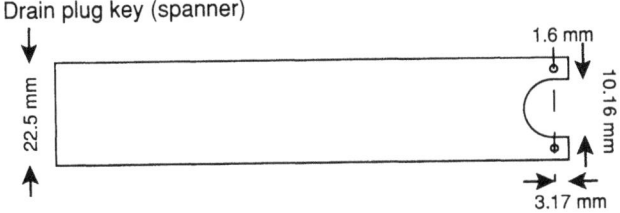

Draw screw

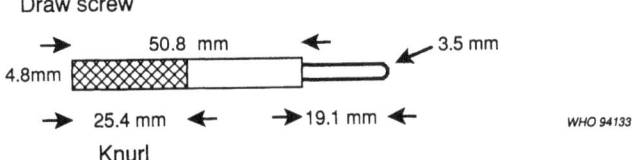

If the manufacturer supplies instructions giving reasons and situations when the equipment should be returned to them or their agent, these should be complied with wherever possible.

Epstein-Macintosh-Oxford (EMO)

The Epstein-Macintosh-Oxford (EMO) (Fig. 4.13) is an anaesthetic vaporizer with low internal resistance, for use with ether and air. It has a water-jacket, which helps to keep the internal temperature constant, and a built-in temperature-compensating valve. The EMO has only two moving parts, the concentration rotor and the temperature compensator. These are set in the factory and should not be altered, except in an emergency, and then only after reading the service manual.

Fig. 4.13. EMO vaporizer: (1) inlet port; (2) outlet port; (3) concentration control; (4) water jacket; (5) thermocompensator valve; (6) vaporizing chamber; (7) filling port for water.

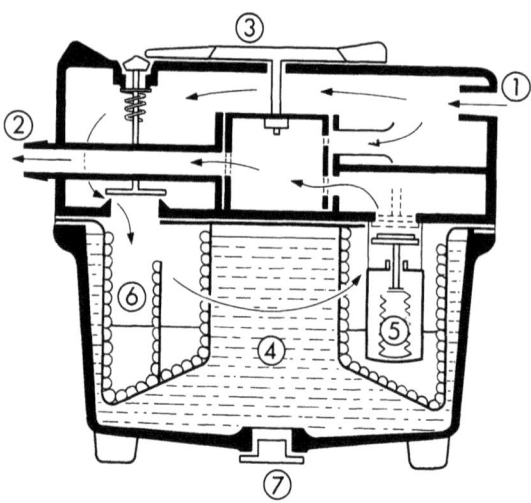

Some simple checks

Level indicator (Fig. 4.14)

With the ether compartment empty, slowly invert the vaporizer and check that the indicator moves freely, falling to the FULL position, and returning to the EMPTY position when the vaporizer is once again upright. When refilling, check that the quantity of ether used complies with the figures given in the instruction book.

Fig. 4.14. EMO: level indicator.

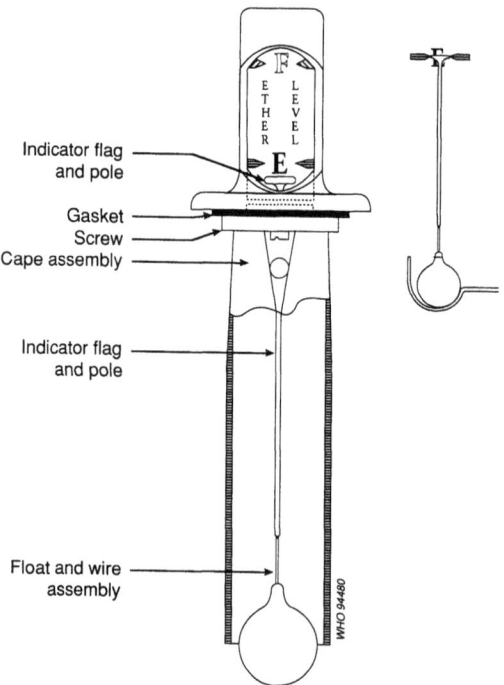

Closing mechanism

Turn the concentration control to the transit position, and connect the outlet of an Oxford inflating bellows, or other ventilating equipment, to the inlet of the EMO. Block the outlet of the EMO, apply gentle pressure to the bellows unit and open the ether filling port. There should be no escape of air through the filling port or through the top of the closing mechanism.

Filling port (Fig. 4.15)

With the bellows still connected to the inlet of the EMO and the outlet blocked, open the control knob to 10, close the filling port, and apply gentle pressure to the bellows; there should be no leakage through the filling port.

Fig. 4.15. EMO: filler unit.

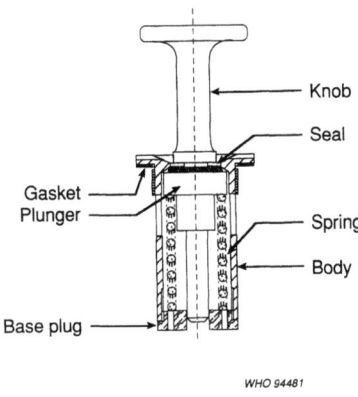

Safety release valve

The safety release valve is combined in the closing mechanism unit. With the control knob set at 2, and with an Oxford bellows connected in the normal position on the outlet of the EMO, block the inlet and check that when the bellows is operated the safety valve operates, drawing air in through the valve.

Temperature compensating unit

The position of the temperature compensating indicator will show whether the unit is in satisfactory working order. The indicator consists of a rod with a black and red band, and a metal top. At 20–25 °C, the metal top and black band should be visible. At temperatures above 32 °C, the red band will begin to show. If only the metal can be seen at 20–25 °C, the compensating unit is faulty and should be replaced.

Water compartment

If the water used to fill the water compartment is thought to contain high concentrations of salts or chlorine, it is advisable to empty and refill the compartment from time to time.

Cleaning and sterilizing

Antiseptic solutions should not be used for cleaning the inhaler. The exterior may be cleaned by wiping with a cloth damped in ether. Sterilizing is not normally necessary as the inhaler is used on open circuit, and protected from contamination by non-return valves. If special circumstances make it necessary to sterilize the instrument, the only suitable method is by the use of ethylene dioxide gas. Excessive heat, such as during boiling or autoclaving, would damage the inhaler.

Fault-finding and rectification

In the event of difficulties in service read the manufacturer's instruction manual carefully. The following notes provide sufficient information for the user to obtain the best possible service from the EMO. It must be stressed that only pure ether should be used in the ether EMO; impurities may cause serious corrosion.

The causes of some of the commoner faults are listed in Table 4.1.

Table 4.1. Common faults with the EMO vaporizer

Fault	Cause	Rectification by user
Concentration control seized	Rotor seized	Return EMO to service engineer or agent
Ether escaping, although control is in "closed for transit" position	Broken level-indicator glass	Replace level-indicator unit
	Broken indicator glass on temperature compensating unit	Replace temperature compensating unit
	Closing mechanism not shutting	Adjust or replace closing-mechanism unit
Concentrations appear to be higher than normal initially, but drop rapidly during use	Temperature compensator not operating	Check the temperature compensating unit and replace if necessary
	Filling port left open	Close filling port
Concentrations appear to be lower than normal	Leak in circuit	Find and rectify
	Relief valve on closing mechanism stuck open	Check the safety release valve. Replace closing mechanism unit, if necessary
	Overfilled with ether so that vaporizing surface area is too small	Pour out excess ether and check level-indicator.
	Temperature compensator not operating	Check the temperature compensating unit; if it is suspect replace it
Level indicator fails to rise when ether is added, but moves freely when inhaler is inverted	Broken float	Replace level-indicator unit.
Level indicator sticks at any point and will not move when inhaler is inverted	Float caught by frayed wick	Remove unit, cut away frayed ends of wicks with scissors.
	Caught by collapsed ether compartment, owing to gas build-up in water jacket due to use of impure water.	Return to makers or agent for servicing

Replace defective parts in all cases. Spare parts are readily available from the manufacturer or from the principal agents, some on a service/exchange basis. This arrangement means that the defective part is returned to the firm, and a new or reconditioned one sent in exchange. When ordering spare parts, the serial number of the inhaler should be given, and the defective part returned with the order.

Fitting a new glass float

1. The wire on the glass float is crimped into a tubular form. To release the old wire, squeeze the tube across the direction of crimping, and pull the wire out with a straight pull.
2. Insert the wire on the new float, and crimp the tube lightly with a pair of pliers.
3. Fit the level-indicator assembly into the empty EMO inhaler, and check the position of the indicator when the float is resting on the bottom of the ether chamber. Adjust, so that the indicator is level with the two arrows on either side of 'E', by pulling or pushing the float as required.
4. When the position is satisfactory, crimp the tube in a second place more heavily to secure the float wire.

Temperature compensating unit (Fig. 4.16)

When ordering a replacement unit, specify the part number and the serial number of the inhaler marked on a plate on the back of the body.

Fig. 4.16. EMO: temperature compensating unit.

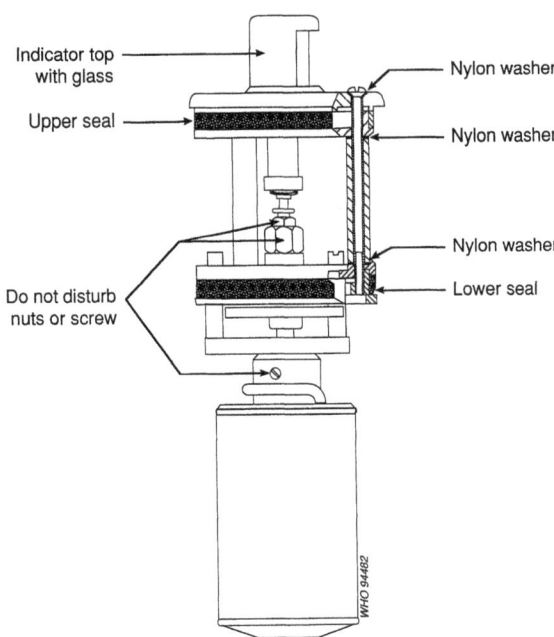

The unit is retained in the inhaler by three screws which expand rubber sealing sleeves when tightened. To remove the old unit:

1. Slacken all the screws by 3–4 turns.
2. Tap the heads of the screws down flush, using a plastic or wooden block.
3. Grip the top of the unit and twist or wriggle it slightly to break the grip of the rubber seals. You should then be able to lift out the unit.

It may be necessary to repeat steps 1 and 2 if the inhaler has been in use for some time. Do not remove the screws completely, as parts may be lost inside the inhaler. If the screws fall into the inhaler, they may be retrieved by tipping the machine up.

To fit a new unit:

1. Make sure that the well in the inhaler body is clean. Slacken the three screws, and slide the unit into the inhaler body.
2. Check that the top plate fits correctly to the inhaler, without gaps, and tighten the screws.

Note: If the unit is removed for any reason, it is desirable to fit new rubber seals before it is refitted into the inhaler. These are available as: lower sealing ring, upper sealing ring, and nylon washers for screw heads. EMO inhalers made after January 1986 have O-ring seals that replace the lower and upper sealing rings.

Closing mechanism (Fig. 4.17)

The closing mechanism unit is retained in the inhaler by two "dogs" operated by screws (marked A in Fig. 4.17). To release the unit, unscrew these by 2 or 3 turns only, and tap the top of the unit lightly with a piece of wood or plastic to break the grip of the sealing washer. A further turn on each screw should then release the dogs and the complete unit can be lifted out.

Fig. 4.17. EMO: closing mechanism.

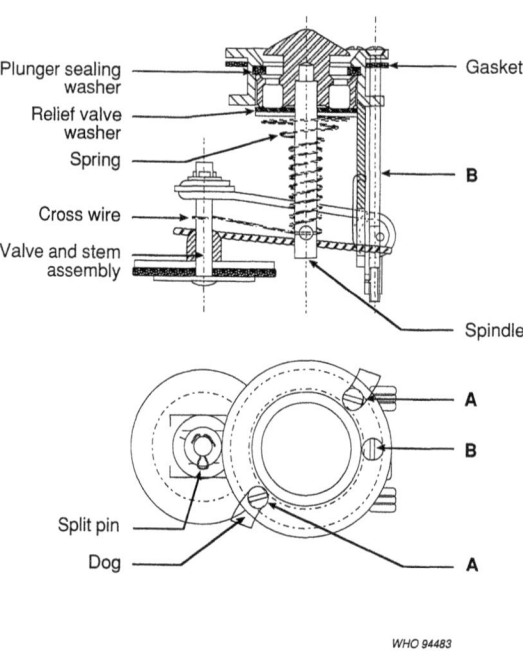

To reattach the closing mechanism to the inhaler, make sure that the dogs are turned fully in, and insert the unit into its seating, checking that the tongue provided on the inhaler fits into the slot in the body of the closing mechanism.

Tighten the two screws by one turn, lift the unit to check that both dogs are engaged and then tighten the screws fully.

To fit a new valve assembly:

1. Remove the split pin and small washer. Discard the split pin.
2. Using fine pliers, disengage the spring wire from the hole in the valve stem.
3. Remove the whole valve-stem assembly and fit a new unit by reversing the procedure. Use a new split pin.

To fit a new relief washer:

1. Pull down the spring, and hold the spindle inside it.
2. By pressing the spindle away from the closing-mechanism body, disengage the top end. The washer can then readily be replaced.

To fit a new body sealing washer:

1. Remove the two screws, 'A', and dogs and adjusting screw, 'B'.
2. Remove the old washer by stretching it over the body. Fit the new washer in the same way.

3. Reassemble dogs and screws 'A' and 'B'.
4. Check against Fig. 4.17 for the correct position. The dogs should be a tight fit on screws 'A'.
5. Readjust unit as described below.

Adjustment of unit fitted to inhaler:

1. After fitting, a new unit may need to be adjusted to ensure correct seating of the valve. Screw 'B' is provided for this purpose. Turning this screw clockwise will increase the closing pressure on the valve.
2. The screw should be adjusted so that the control pointer can operate the closing mechanism without undue force, and the valve closes soundly when checked as described on page 87.

As already stated, the rotor is correctly adjusted before the machine leaves the factory, and should not be interfered with in any way.

Boyle's ether vaporizer

Boyle's ether vaporizer operates through a controllable bypass, which directs the required proportion of anaesthetic gas (0–100%) through a U-tube, to emerge over the liquid ether contained in the glass jar. Vapour concentration may be increased to a maximum by depressing the cowl plunger, thus causing the gas to bubble through the liquid (Fig. 4.18).

Fig. 4.18. Boyle's ether vaporizer.

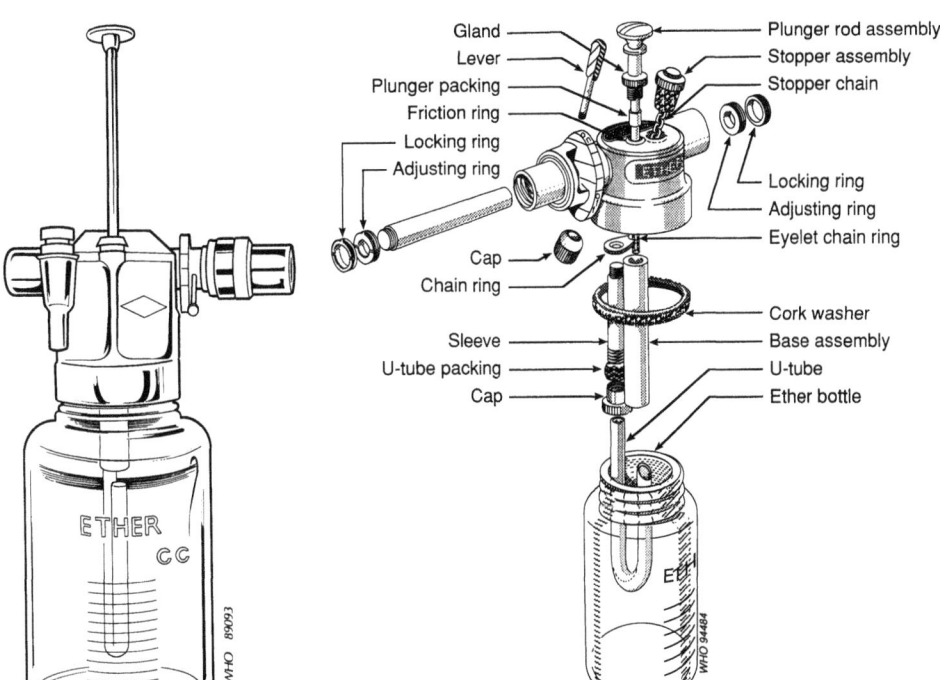

Servicing

Boyle's ether vaporizer should be serviced as follows:

1. Check that all the apparatus gas supplies are turned off.
2. Remove the vaporizer from the back-bar assembly.
3. Remove the locking nut and adjustment rings from the gas-inlet side of the vaporizer body.

4. Remove the drum-actuating lever and withdraw the drum. (If the drum is seized or cannot readily be withdrawn, remove the locking ring from the gas outlet and turn the adjusting ring in a clockwise direction to force the drum out.)
5. Examine the drum for signs of scoring or corrosion; remove the old grease and apply a film of a suitable grease.
6. Remove the drum-grease injector cap and clean all the old grease from the body assembly.
7. Unscrew the plunger-control-gland packing nut, probe out the packing cotton and regrease it. Replace the cotton and the gland-packing nut.
8. Insert the drum and refit the actuating lever.
9. With the outlet-adjusting ring removed, screw in the inlet adjusting ring, while moving the actuating lever to and fro, until an increase in resistance to lever movement is felt. (**Do not** overtighten the ring to the point of drum seizure, as this will force out all the grease.)
10. Without moving the adjusting ring, fit and tighten the inlet locking ring.
11. Screw in the outlet adjusting ring until it just touches the drum, then back off one-eighth of a turn; fit and tighten the locking ring.
12. Check the drum for freedom of operation.
13. Fill the grease-injector cap with grease and screw in to the grease point.
14. Examine the glass bottle for dirt and damage; replace as necessary.
15. Examine the U-tube and cowl for dirt and damage, and for security of attachment.
16. Examine the bottle-sealing washer for serviceability; replace as necessary.
17. Examine the cork stopper for serviceability and security of attachment to the retaining chain.
18. Refit the vaporizer into the back-bar unit assembly.
19. Using a continuity test-set, or multimeter, check that there is electrical continuity between the drum-actuating lever, the cowl-operating plunger, and the vaporizer body.
20. Test the back-bar for leaks. See p. 94 for the back-bar tests.

Testing anaesthetic machines, ventilators and related equipment

Anaesthetic machines and ventilators should be tested in the room or area where the equipment is situated, if at all possible. Service personnel must wear accepted operating-room clothing in the surgical areas.

Contact the person responsible for operating-room equipment regarding the movement or servicing of any such equipment.

Anaesthetic machines

Tools and materials required

Normal service tools
Silicone grease
Light oil[1]
Service manuals
Watch with a second-hand
Spare parts

---

[1] Do not use ordinary oil (such as motor oil) to lubricate any parts that come into contact with oxygen.

Mercury sphygmomanometer
Anaesthetic gas analyser (if available)
Device for measuring flow, pressure and tidal volume

Testing procedure

If there is an official service manual, follow the steps outlined in it; otherwise, follow the procedure below (see Fig. 4.5, page 75).

- Check for leaks in the high-pressure system:
  1. Turn off all flowmeters, and disconnect any ancillary equipment such as ventilators and suckers.
  2. Turn on each cylinder in turn and allow the system to pressurize, then turn the cylinder off. Watch the pressure gauge; if the needle drops, there is a leak.
  3. Remove the covers and brush each joint, or suspect point, with soapy water. Do not forget to check inside the back of the pressure gauge. A leak will be indicated by the formation of bubbles. Do this for each cylinder in turn.

- Check the operation of each flowmeter. Make sure the control knob stays where it is set, and is not liable to be turned by mistake.
  1. Close all valves on the machine. Open all cylinder valves one full turn, noting any movement of the flowmeter floats. Float movement indicates a leaky flowmeter valve. If so, adjust the stop so that gas flow ceases 1/8 turn before the knob reaches the stop.
  2. Verify flowmeter accuracy ($\pm$ 2.5% full scale), with the measuring device connected to the common gas outlet.
  3. Check that the needle-valve stems are tight enough to remain where set unless deliberately turned by the operator.

- Check the low-pressure system, which is the part from the control knobs to the outlet.
  1. Check the top and bottom seals on the flow tubes with a low-pressure test.
     - Connect a mercury sphygmomanometer to the outlet.
     - Turn on the oxygen flowmeter very slowly.
     - Pressurize the back-bar to 30 mmHg (4 kPa). When this pressure is reached turn down the flow until the pressure on the gauge remains constant at 30 mmHg (4 kPa).
     - If the flow is less than 100 ml/min, it is acceptable; if it is greater than this, look for a leak.
  2. Check all the joints on the back-bar with a high-pressure test.
     - Pressurize the system to 150 mmHg (20 kPa).
     - Reduce the flow to maintain that pressure.
     - If the flow is 100 ml/min or less, it is acceptable; if it is greater than this, look for a leak. Brush each suspect point with soapy water; bubbles will appear at the site of the leak.

- Check the correct operation of the oxygen-failure warning whistle (if fitted). Pressurize the intermediate system, turn off the supply, and open the oxygen-flowmeter valve to reduce the pressure slowly. The whistle should sound for a minimum of 10 seconds when the pressure falls to between 180 and 250 kPa. Check that the flow of nitrous oxide is cut off when the oxygen is turned off (if that system is fitted).
- Check the oxygen-flush valve. It should allow a flow greater than 35 litres/min, but not more than 75 litres/min (or as required by local regulations).

- If there are hoses for connection to a wall supply, check these. Check the oxygen flow from the oxygen flow tube when the oxygen probe is plugged in and the nitrous oxide disconnected. Similarly, when the nitrous oxide probe is plugged in and the oxygen disconnected, nitrous oxide must flow from the nitrous oxide flow tube, and nothing from the oxygen flow tube.
- Check the non-return valve on each of the yokes. Pressurize the system, turn off the cylinder, and remove it. There should be no gas leak. If there is a leak, look for the simple non-return valve in the yoke. Dismantle and clean the valve, then reassemble.
- If the anaesthetist has been having difficulty in getting patients to sleep, or waking them up, there may be a problem with the vaporizer. Inspect the mountings and connectors to ensure that they are secure and leak-free. When servicing vaporizers, be sure to keep them in an upright position when they contain liquid anaesthetic. To check the vaporizer, an anaesthetic gas analyser is required. Connect the gas analyser to the common gas outlet. Set the oxygen flow to 3 litres/min, and after zeroing the gas analyser with 100% oxygen, test each vaporizer at each full percentage setting. Determine that there is no concentration of gas when the vaporizers are in the "off" position. Replace any vaporizer for which the concentration is incorrect by more than 0.3% of the reading, or 10% of the measured value, whichever is greater. If an anaesthetic gas analyser is not available, you can only check (a) that the vaporizer is off when it is turned off, (b) that it gives an output when it is turned on again, and (c) that the concentration of gas increases as the control is turned up.

  Check that the control knob turns smoothly. Vaporizers should be returned to the manufacturers, or their agents, for checking every few years. The interval depends upon the model; some models need a check by the company only every 10 years.
- Check the smooth operation of the pressure gauges. The pointer should move smoothly and come to rest before the flow in the flow tube stops. If the movement is not smooth, lubricate the linkage in the back with silicone grease.
- Check the absorber. Check for smooth operation of the controls and for leaks. Change the filling if required.
- Check any other back-bar-mounted equipment.
- Check the output pressure of the regulators. This should be around 390 kPa (or as required by local regulations), and in any case should be about 35 kPa lower than the output pressure from the wall outlet.
- Check all flexible tubing on the machine.
- Check all attached equipment, such as suckers and blood pressure machines.
- Check the drawers, wheels, and the general frame of the machine. Lubricate lightly as required.
- Clean the machine.
- Tick off all tests on the service sheet, and sign it.
- Return the machine to the user. The doctor in charge should test it to make sure that it operates satisfactorily.

Ventilators

Tools and materials required

Normal service tools
Silicone grease
Light oil
Service manuals (if available)
Watch with a second-hand
Spare parts (if available)
Device for measuring flow, pressure and tidal volume

Testing procedure

It is of the utmost importance that all ventilators should work safely, since lives depend upon their correct operation. In addition, ventilators should **never** be used without a correctly adjusted alarm system, which gives a warning, and therefore protects the patient, in case of malfunction or disconnection.

If you do not have the service manual for your machine, make every effort to get one. Make sure a service manual is ordered with every new machine. Even without the manual, it is still possible to ensure that the machine is working correctly, but the proper spare parts must be available. Records are very important when maintaining ventilators and other life-support equipment. All reported faults, repairs, and service details should be noted down, dated, and signed. Machines should be serviced twice a year.

If you are called to look at a machine that has been reported as faulty, check first that it has been set up properly. Most reported faults are caused by operator error. When looking for a fault, start from the beginning. For example, is the electricity turned on? Is the gas on? Investigate the device in a planned manner, looking for the obvious things first. If you have doubts about the machine's safety or correct operation and you are unable to repair it on the spot, take it out of service. If there is no spare machine, the patient must be ventilated with a resuscitation bag while the machine is being repaired.

If it is not possible to repair a machine properly owing to a lack of spare parts, do not be tempted to carry out temporary repairs. Report the problem to the user, ask for the spares, and remove the machine from use.

Do not agree to put a machine back into service against your better judgement. If the personnel on the ward insist, get them to sign the service sheet (with the problem clearly stated).

Follow the steps outlined in the official service book. To carry out a service without the book, follow the steps outlined below:

1. Inspect the outside of the machine, including all tubing, connectors, and any bellows for damage. Replace as required. Lightly rub any antistatic tubing, or bellows, with silicone grease to prevent perishing.
2. Connect up to the electricity and gas supplies, as required. Put a stopper or test lung on the patient connector and start the machine running. Set the controls to normal settings. Watch that the operation is regular and smooth. Listen and check for any unusual noises. It is important to use the same regular settings in each test; in this way, you will get to know the normal movements and sounds of correct operation. Any unusual movements or sounds will alert you to possible problems.
3. Switch off and disconnect the machine from the mains. Remove the covers. Inspect any internal tubing or bellows, lightly rub any antistatic tubing or bellows with silicone grease to prevent perishing. Replace as required. Blow clean, and wipe the insides. If there are electronic circuit boards, check that they are secure and show no damage. Check for wear in any moving mechanical parts. Using a light motor oil, or similar, lightly lubricate any moving pivot points. Clean up any drips.
4. Start the machine running again, taking care not to touch any internal parts; watch any internal movements (bellows, lever, or valve movements) for smooth operation.
5. Try each control in turn and check that it does what is intended; for example, if the breath-rate control says that the machine will do 60 breaths per minute, this must be confirmed. With all these checks, a degree of common sense is

necessary. For example, do not worry if the breath-rate control says 60 and only 58 are delivered. Every machine has a margin of error. If the manual is not available, a degree of discretion should be used.
6. Check that the pressure gauge is accurate by comparing it with a test gauge.
7. Check the correct operation of all lights and indicators.
8. To check the correct operation of the oxygen mixer, an oxygen analyser is needed. If your department does not have one, ask the Anaesthetic Department to provide such an instrument. Note down on the service sheet the output results from 21% to 100%.
9. Check the alarm system.
10. Run the machine again on the normal settings and check that it is still working correctly.
11. If it is a machine that uses electricity, give it a safety check.
12. Fill out the service check-sheet, and sign it.

As you gain more experience in servicing, you will get to know which errors are minor, and can be allowed, and which are unacceptable. For example, an oxygen mixer on a paediatric ventilator **must not** give higher levels of inspired oxygen than indicated. This is because very serious damage can be done to the infant's eyes as a result.

Return the machine to the user; the doctor in charge should test it to ensure that it operates satisfactorily.

Ventilator bellows

Mechanical integrity

Inspect the bellows housing and base for cracks, chips, etc. Check the tubing and control knobs for tightness.

Over-pressure valve

Check the valve, located on the scavenging tee at the back of the control unit, for cleanliness and operation.

Pop-off valve

Remove the housing, bellows, and pop-off valve from the base. Check that the pop-off valve, glass disc, and seat are clean and dry, and that the retaining screw is tight.

Bellows flexibility

Reassemble the ventilator and connect the test gauge to the common gas outlet. Inflate the bellows to 0.1 litre. If the pressure is above 1.75 cm water (1.3 mm Hg) then the bellows should be replaced.

Bellows pressure (low)

Connect the device for measuring pressure to the common gas outlet, open the oxygen flowmeter to 300 ml/min, and allow the bellows to rise to the top. The pressure should be less than 2.5 cm water (1.84 mm Hg or equivalent on the gauge in use), and the bellows should remain full. If the bellows do not remain up, or the pressure exceeds 2.5 cm water, then refer to the ventilator service manual for the necessary repairs.

Bellows pressure (high)

Connect the common gas outlet to the driving gas port on the bellows, and plug the bellows outlet. Pressurize the outside of the bellows to just above 60 cm water

(44 mm Hg) and maintain an oxygen flow of 300 ml/min. The pressure gauge should settle at or above 60 cm water. If the pressure drops below 60 cm water, refer to the ventilator service manual for the necessary repairs.

Ventilator controller

Low-oxygen-supply alarm

Check that the low-oxygen alarm activates before the supply pressure to the ventilator drops below 250 kPa, and resets when the pressure reaches 320 kPa.

Low-airway-pressure alarm

Check that the alarm activates if the pressure measured at the patient port remains below 7 cm water (5 mm Hg or equivalent on the gauge in use) for between 20 and 30 seconds.

Safety valve

Check that the relief valve opens when the pressure in the patient circuit exceeds 65–75 cm water (48–55 mmHg or equivalent on the gauge in use).

Flow delivery

Set the ventilator as follows:

minute volume	10
rate	10
inspiratory: expiratory (I:E) ratio	1:1

Start the ventilator; the tidal volume measured with a spirometer, or ventilator tester, should be between 0.9 and 1.1 litres/min. If it is not, first check the rate with a stopwatch and adjust if necessary. Check the I:E ratio with a stopwatch at a very low rate, and adjust if necessary. After confirming that both are correct, reset the ventilator to the above settings and adjust the minute volume to give a 1 litre tidal volume.

Absorbers

Canister

Check for cracks and chips, and check gaskets. Replace as necessary.

Inspiratory and expiratory valves

Inspect the inspiratory and expiratory valves for cleanliness, and for bent or chipped discs.

Bag/ventilator switch (if fitted)

Inspect the valve, clean, and lubricate with silicone grease, as necessary, to maintain free action.

Relief valve

Inspect, clean, and lubricate screw-threads with silicone grease. Check that when the valve is fully open a maximum pressure of 0.3 kPa (2.5 mm Hg) is maintained in the system with the oxygen flowmeter opened to flood measured with the device for measuring flow, pressure and tidal volume at the bag connector.

Drain valve

Inspect and clean as necessary.

Elevating assembly

Check that the push-button operates smoothly; raise and lower the assembly several times to check operation. If it does not operate smoothly, disassemble and clean with alcohol. **Do not lubricate**.

Compound pressure gauge

Test the patient pressure gauge for zero setting and accuracy ($\pm 5\%$ of reading) with the pressure-measuring device attached to the bag connector. Calibrate, if necessary, with the adjusting screw located under the plug-screw, inside the absorber head, beneath the screen.

Pressure regulators (reducing valves) and flowmeters

The pressure regulator, or reducing valve, as the name suggests, is used to reduce the pressure of a gas from the cylinder pressure to a pressure that is safe for subsequent delivery to a patient. For example, in the case of oxygen, it is from 14 300 to 420 kPa. A flowmeter can be attached to the regulator to allow a given flow to be set. These assemblies are most common on anaesthetic machines, or on an oxygen therapy unit attached to the top of a gas cylinder.

When used in oxygen therapy[1], there are three parts to the unit:
- a gauge showing the pressure of the contents of the cylinder,
- a regulator to reduce the pressure,
- a flowmeter that indicates the selected flow.

There are a number of different designs of regulator, but generally each unit has one inlet (from the cylinder) and three outlets, one to the pressure gauge, one to the flowmeter, and one to the blow-off valve. It is important to know which one is meant to be connected to the pressure gauge: do not connect any other part to this outlet.

While the proper checking of pressure regulators requires some special test equipment, most problems can be overcome with very little equipment.

Remember that the flow tube is under regulator pressure. Do not unscrew it before the cylinder is turned off and the pressure released.

Setting the output pressure

Make sure that the cylinder contents gauge and the safety valve are connected to the regulator, remove the flowmeter and fit in its place a 0–700 kPa pressure gauge. Connect the regulator to the gas cylinder, and turn on the gas. The test pressure gauge should show a reading of 420 kPa. This is the correct pressure for an oxygen therapy regulator and flowmeter. If it is not 420 kPa, adjust with a socket head key until it is correct. If you are adjusting the pressure downwards, you must release the pressure from the test gauge, turn the adjusting screw out,

---

[1] Do not use any oil when repairing oxygen regulators. If you use PTFE or plumbers' tape, you should use only special de-greased tape.

reconnect the test gauge, and adjust the pressure up to 420 kPa. On most makes, the adjustment screw will be found at the end of the piece which sticks out at the front; it may be covered with a sticky label.

At this pressure, it should be possible to obtain a flow of up to 55 litres/min out of the unit; this is called the flush flow. In some places, the regulator is not set for pressure but adjusted for a given flow with the control wide open; check what is required before adjusting the setting.

For a regulator attached to an anaesthetic machine, adjust the pressure to about 390 kPa (30 kPa lower than the pressure from the pipeline supply to the machine).

Testing a regulator and flowmeter unit

1. Check for leaks.
2. Check that the pointer on the gauge works smoothly and reaches the stop before the flow falls to zero.
3. Check that the flow goes to its full rate.

Faults

- If a leak is suspected, check as follows:
    - With the flowmeter unit turned off, turn on the gas and allow the pressure to rise. Turn off the gas supply.
    - The system is now pressurized to the full cylinder pressure, but with a very small volume.
    - If there is any leak, the gauge will show a fall in pressure; the bigger the leak the faster the fall.
    - If the pressure falls, brush the unit with soapy water; any leaks will show up as small bubbles.
    - Do not forget to check inside the back of the gauge.

- Leaks around the bull-nose connector are usually caused by a faulty O-ring. Replace the ring.
- Leaks at the blow-off valve:
    - First, check that the regulator is set to the correct output pressure.
    - If the pressure rises to more than it should, yet the regulator is set to the correct output pressure, there is a faulty valve seat (a problem called "creep"). Replace the valve seat.

    The blow-off valve should normally go off at about 640 kPa.

- If the flowmeter makes a popping noise when the flow is turned on ("motor boating"), there is probably dirt inside the valve; the noise may also be caused by a faulty valve seat.
- Low flows: unscrew the needle valve and check that it is clean and undamaged.
- If the ball, or bobbin, shows a small flow even when the unit is turned off, check the flow tube for leaks.
- If the gauge needle does not drop smoothly, remove the back of the gauge and lubricate the movement of the gauge with a light watch oil. Use of oil is acceptable in this case, as there is no oxygen flowing in this part.
- If there is no flow, even when the gauge shows that there is gas in the cylinder, this suggests that the gauge needle is stuck. Check the movement in the back of the gauge, or reposition the needle on the shaft.

Unregulated flowmeters, in which the flowmeter is connected directly to the gas cylinder, are dangerous and should not be used.

Oxygen analysers

Inspection and calibration

Visually inspect the cables and the display unit for signs of wear or deterioration. Check that the sensor membrane is not nicked or otherwise damaged, and that the O-ring seal is intact. Test the calibration by first placing the sensor in a T-adaptor, in a verified 100% oxygen line, and allow the readings to stabilize. If, after 3 minutes, the display has not stabilized, replace the sensor. If it has stabilized, adjust the CAL knob, if necessary, so that the display registers 100%. Remove the sensor from the T-adaptor and expose to room air. A reading of 21% ($\pm$ 2%) should be displayed within 1 minute. If a correct reading is not displayed, replace the sensor.

5. Operation room equipment

Antistatic equipment and apparatus

Precautions need to be taken against the build-up of static electricity to avoid creating a risk of explosion. The risk of electrostatic ignition is particularly high in the immediate surroundings of anaesthetic apparatus and its attachments. Flammable gas mixtures escaping from the anaesthetic breathing circuits are rapidly diluted to a nonflammable level within a few centimetres of the point of escape. The zone of risk associated with flammable anaesthetics is now recognized as extending for 25 cm around any part of the anaesthetic circuit, or of the gas pathways of an anaesthetic apparatus. All portable equipment that is liable to be located within this zone when the anaesthetic apparatus is in use should be antistatic. In addition to eliminating electrostatic materials on such equipment, all metallic parts should be continuous and have an effective antistatic contact with the floor, e.g., by being fitted with antistatic castors. Although the electrostatic risk can be eliminated for a period by applying an antistatic polish to exposed surfaces of plastic parts, it must be remembered that these polishes (which are often water-soluble) are liable to be washed off when the equipment is cleaned, or to be rubbed off during use.

Oxygen alone is not flammable and, while it is possible to ignite fibres contaminated with oil or grease by an electrostatic spark in an oxygen-enriched atmosphere, the risk is small in places such as oxygen tents, unless a flammable gas or vapour is present.

Humidity

High humidity helps combat static electricity. The thin film of water on equipment conducts the static away. But humidity alone cannot be relied upon as an antistatic precaution. A humidifier is liable to fail, and the degree of humidification necessary may be difficult to achieve in very dry conditions. Also, high relative humidity may be uncomfortable for the staff. Humidity is much less effective as an antistatic measure with most plastics and with fabrics that tend to be moisture-repellent. With good antistatic precautions, low humidity does not create a risk, provided the materials do not lose their antistatic properties.

Requirements for antistatic materials, and antistatic tests

The resistance of rubber used for patient tubes, trolley wheels, and other items requiring antistatic properties may need to be checked periodically. Some examples of levels of resistance for various antistatic items (as recommended in the United Kingdom) are listed below:

– antistatic tubing forming the main connection between the patient and an anaesthetic machine: 25 000 ohms minimum, 1 megohm maximum;
– mattresses and pads: 5000 ohms minimum, 1 megohm maximum;
– fabrics: 50 000 ohms minimum, 100 000 megohms maximum;
– footwear: 50 000 ohms minimum, 50 megohms maximum;
– castor tyres: no lower limit, 1 megohm maximum.

The resistance of some antistatic materials may increase with age and use. The recommended upper limit for all equipment in service is 100 megohms. If the resistance rises above this it is considered to have lost its antistatic properties and may have to be withdrawn from use.

Antistatic rubber should be marked with a yellow line and be printed with the word "antistatic" where it is practical to do so. The instrument recommended for testing antistatic properties is an insulation tester, having an open-circuit voltage of about 500 volts DC. A typical insulation tester has a voltage characteristic such that the voltage falls as the test resistance falls. Significant errors may occur if the voltage across the test resistance falls below 40 volts DC.

Test method

For most of the tests, small test clips are used as electrodes. When testing flat surfaces, use clean metal electrodes having a flat surface of about 625 mm². Select, and wet, two areas, each of approximately 625 mm² (25 mm × 25 mm), on the item to be tested, the test area being chosen so that the result represents the resistance of the longest discharge path through the article. Where difficulty is experienced in wetting the surface, e.g., of rubber, a wetting agent, such as detergent, should be added to the water. The test areas will usually be at the extreme opposite ends, e.g., of tubing and breathing bags, or on the top and bottom surfaces of pads and mattresses. On thin sheeting, the test areas should be on the same surface with about 50 mm of dry surface between them. Both surfaces of thin sheeting should be tested. (Measurements made through the thickness of thin sheeting are unreliable, as they can be influenced by small isolated areas of conductivity.)

For trolley castor tyres, test for continuity between the metal frame of the trolley and the tyre, in addition to measuring the resistance of the tyre. A convenient method for testing trolley tyres is to stand the tyre on a wetted metal plate which is insulated from the floor, e.g., on a piece of rubber sheeting. Make the test between the metal plate and the metal parts of the trolley.

For footwear, one of the electrodes should be placed on a surface that will be in close contact with the wearer and the other on the surface that will be in contact with the floor, when the footwear is in use.

Operating table

An operating table is more than just a table for the surgeon to operate on; it must be possible to adjust it up and down, to tilt the head up and down, and to move it to suit the needs of the operation. As the tables are often very heavy, most of them have wheels and a brake, so that they can be moved about the room. On each side, there is a rail to which clamps can be fastened to hold various attachments as required, for example for the lithotomy position. The antistatic mattresses are filled with foam and have a number of separate sections.

In the older types of operating table, the table is positioned by turning a large knob by hand. With this type, maintenance is fairly simple and limited to keeping the threads of the screws lubricated, and the mattresses in good order. The adjustments will probably work for several years without need of attention.

To prevent the mattresses perishing, apply a little silicone grease to the rubber cover. Check for splits in the rubber covering and repair as necessary. This is important, since such splits allow entry of moisture and particulate matter into the foam and predispose to the growth of bacteria. Simple tears and splits in rubber covers should be repaired using patches and rubber glue, of the type used for the repair of bicycle inner-tubes. To repair a small hole, use glue and a suitable patch. Clean the area to be patched. Rub around the area of the hole with fine sandpaper to roughen the surface a little. Clean off any dust or grit left from the sandpaper and apply the glue to the area to be covered by the patch. Allow this to dry until the glue no longer feels tacky. Apply the patch and press it down well, then apply a weight over a flat object placed on the repaired area. Leave it for a while. Remove the weight and the flat object. The patch should have stuck.

Other operating tables are of the hydraulic type, movement being achieved by pumping a pedal to move the parts hydraulically, as with a car jack. With these tables the hydraulic oil is likely to leak when the seals around the pistons become worn or perished. Although it may be possible to pump the table up, it may not stay at the required level. This is caused by a leak in the release mechanism, allowing oil to seep back. A motor mechanic who repairs hydraulic jacks may be able to help in solving this problem, and may even have seals that will fit the table. The hydraulic oil will certainly be similar. Alternatively, contact the manufacturer of the operating table. A label giving the manufacturer's name and address is likely to be on the table. Explain the problem and ask for advice in resolving it. Ask for a service manual at the same time.

It is important to remember that hydraulic tables can be repaired without expensive spares, even if it means resorting to the motor trade.

Suction apparatus

The usual atmospheric pressure used for calibration is 760 mmHg (100 kPa or 14.7 psi), which is the standard at sea level. Negative pressure is any pressure that is less than atmospheric, or zero, on the pressure gauge. A vacuum force can thus be described as a negative pressure; suction is the application of that negative pressure, and relates to the movement of gas, fluids, or solids so caused.

Negative pressure can be measured by the amount of vacuum force acting on a given area to lift liquid up a column to a given height. It is generally measured as the height of either mercury or water in inches, centimetres, or millimetres. Mercury and water pressure levels may be marked on the same gauge. A water column, being 13.6 times longer than that of mercury to support the same pressure, is more sensitive. Therefore gauges calibrated with a water column generally cover a smaller range of pressures than those calibrated with a mercury column. A negative pressure equal to 1 mmHg means the amount of vacuum required to lift mercury up a column by 1 millimetre. The same negative pressure will lift water up a column to a height of 13.6 millimetres.

The four main types of suction machine used in hospital practice are described below.

The electric suction machine

This machine has an electric pump which evacuates a bottle (reservoir), to which is attached a suction tube (Fig. 5.1). The system incorporates a pressure gauge and a mechanism to facilitate regulation of the vacuum, by allowing air to be drawn in from the room.

Wall-supplied suction

This normally works in the same way as the electric suction machine, the difference being that the motor generating the suction is some way away, and is connected to several outlets. This type of suction therefore requires a much larger reservoir since more than one outlet may be in use at one time. The wall suction equipment

Fig. 5.1. Electric suction machine.

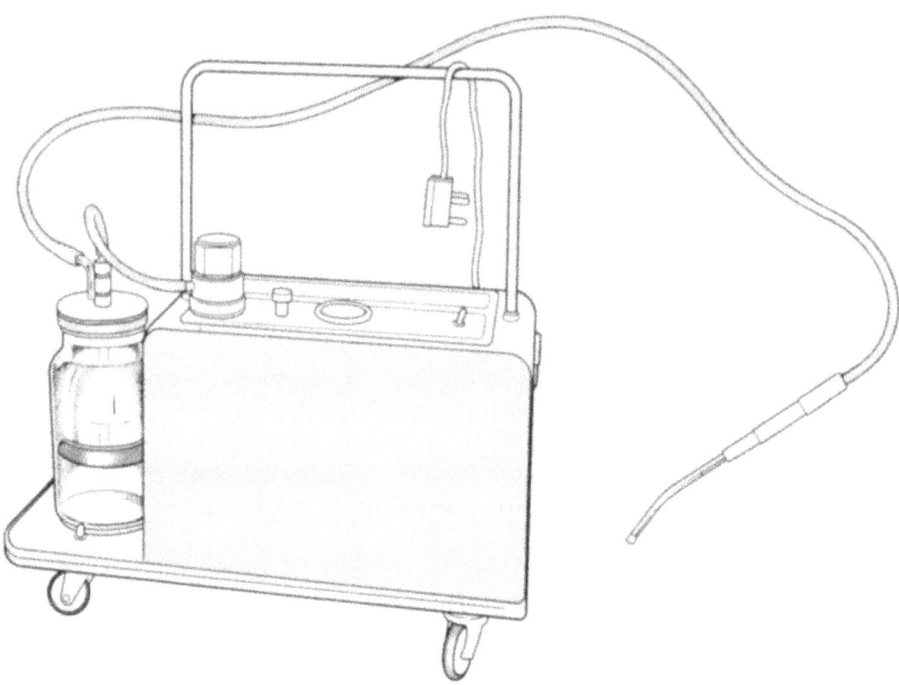

includes a large tank that is evacuated by a pump and to which the suction line is connected. The tank is fitted with a pressure switch that automatically turns on the pump if the vacuum falls below a certain level.

Most suction equipment has a device for regulating the level of vacuum, such as a simple bleed-off screw, or a spring-operated device, that keeps the vacuum at the set level. The wall suction systems often have high and low settings, the latter often being used for infants and children. Modern systems are calibrated in kPa (kilopascals); a low vacuum is up to about 30 kPa, and a high vacuum may be up to about 100 kPa. Other units such as mmHg may be found. Conversion factors for many of these are given in Annex 4.

Foot-operated suction unit

This is the simplest type of suction unit and is operated by pressing on a piston with the foot (Fig. 5.2). On the return stroke of the piston (operated by a spring), suction is created, and a series of valves directs the flow as required. The maintenance of such a suction unit is fairly simple and often only involves making sure that the one-way valves are working correctly, and that there are no leaks in the system.

Piston pumps

These suction pumps have two pistons that are operated by an induction motor, with each piston sucking in turn. The suction line is taken from a bottle connected to the unit, which incorporates a pressure gauge and a pressure-relief valve, so that it can be regulated to the desired pressure. These pumps have only a small capacity, and are used mainly for drainage during surgery. Maintenance involves keeping the unit well oiled; if this is not done, the pump will stop or operate very slowly.

Fig. 5.2. Foot-operated suction machine.

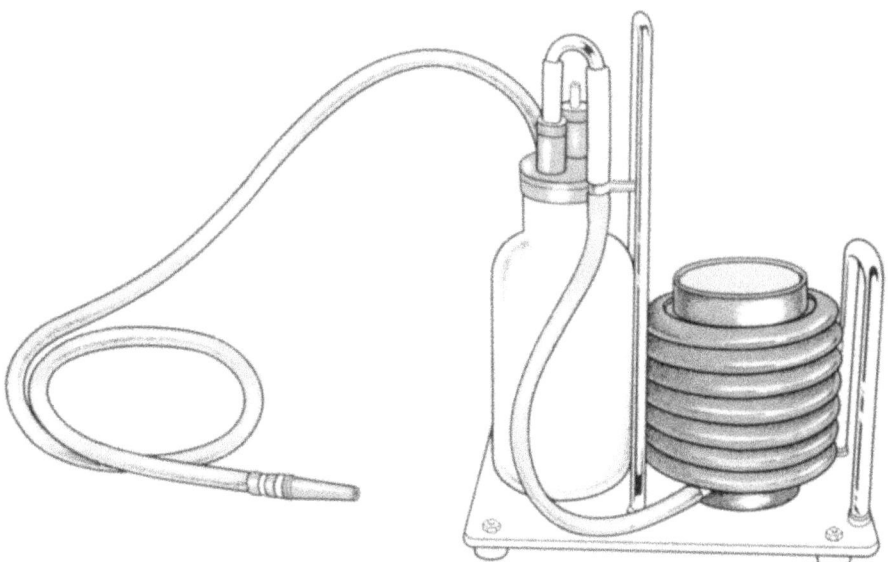

Maintenance and repair

To avoid the possibility of infection, make sure that the machine has been sterilized before starting to work on it; do not put any parts in your mouth, and wash your hands afterwards. **Do not** suck or blow into any part of the machine, and handle all parts with care. Cover any cuts or abrasions, and wear a pair of gloves.

Maintenance of suction systems is for the most part not difficult. The commonly used colour code for a vacuum hose is yellow. Get to know the level of suction to be expected from a unit. Lower levels will indicate a problem somewhere in the system. The most common problem is a leak, which may be in the tubes or inside the machine. It may be that the bottle is not screwed in place properly. Check the sealing washer, and check that the bottle itself is not cracked. To check the bottle and its tubing, remove the tubing where it comes out from the machine and put a finger over the end with the machine turned on. The pressure gauge should go to its maximum. If it does not, then there is a problem inside the machine itself. If it does, the problem is with the bottle or the tubes.

If the problem appears to be inside the machine, take off the covers. If the tubing is not at fault and is tight on the connectors, and if the pressure gauge is working properly, then the fault must lie with the motor. Dismantle the motor in an attempt to locate the problem. A likely cause is a hole in the rubber diaphragm (if it is a diaphragm pump).

If a high vacuum is recorded on the gauge with none at the suction tube, this is usually caused by a blockage in the system.

Surgical diathermy machine

In surgical diathermy, a high-frequency electric current (0.5–2 MHz) is used to produce heat to seal (by coagulation) blood vessels, or to cut and seal at the same time. The heating can be regulated by a variable resistance.

There are two types of diathermy machine: monopolar and bipolar.

In monopolar machines, the current flows from the active electrode through body tissue, along the line of least resistance, to a large indifferent plate electrode and back to the machine. Different waveforms can be used to produce a cutting or coagulating mode. For the cutting mode, the waveform is continuous, while for the coagulating mode, the energy is produced in bursts.

With bipolar diathermy, the two tips of a pair of forceps are the two electrodes; there is no plate electrode. Coagulation occurs when the forceps are closed across a piece of tissue. This technique is very good for dealing with very small blood vessels. The energy output required is low.

Diathermy machines can be classified according to the type of output connection used. The different types are:

- isolated output (Fig. 5.3A);
- radiofrequency earthed output (Fig. 5.3B);
- hard-earthed output (Fig. 5.3C).

Fig. 5.3. Three types of diathermy machine.

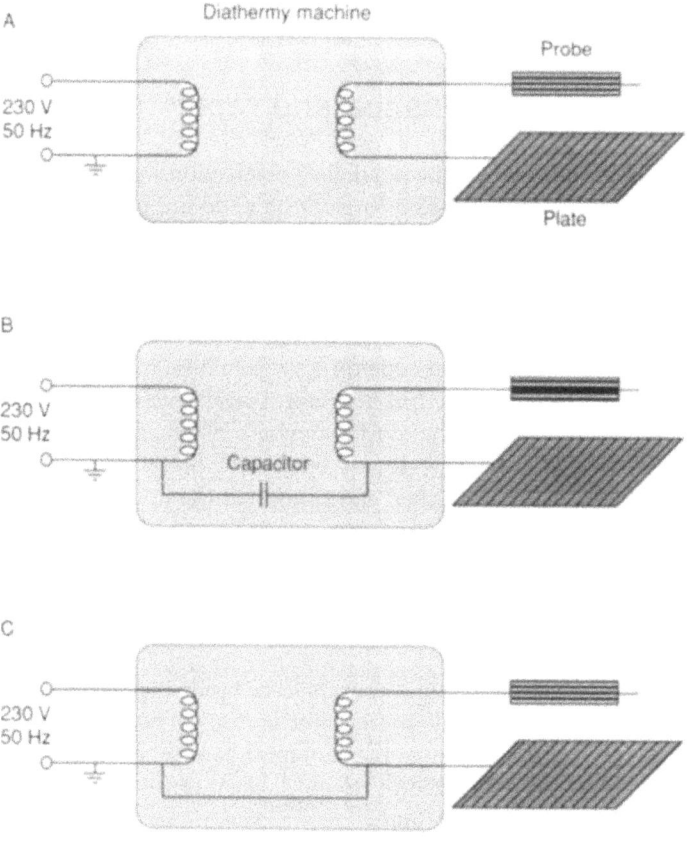

Isolated output machines have both sides of the output floating with respect to earth. This minimizes the risk of possible alternative pathways for radiofrequency current (which can cause burns), or for mains frequency current from the machine itself (which can electrocute).

Radiofrequency earthed output machines have a capacitor placed between the plate side of the output and earth. This permits radiofrequency current to flow to earth. The small value of the capacitor prevents the passage of mains frequency current so that isolation is effectively preserved at the mains frequency; the risks of electrocution are not increased by this method. However, the risk of possible alternative pathways for radiofrequency current to cause burns is greatly increased, and for this reason a plate current monitor is required on such machines. This monitor senses any difference in current flows between the active and the plate leads, and turns off the output if a difference occurs. The difference represents the leakage current.

Hard-earthed output machines have a plate electrode directly connected to earth, so the patient is also directly connected to earth. This means that the risk of electrocution is very much higher. For this reason machines of this design are no longer produced, and any that are still in use should be replaced.

Maintenance

The routine maintenance needed for these machines is limited. Proper records should be kept of all work done on them. Make a check-sheet of work to be done, and then make routine inspections at least twice a year.

The most important job is the electrical safety check. If you do not have an electrical safety checker, follow the instructions in the section on cardiac monitors (pages 67–69). Keep the inside and the outside of the machine clean. Check the plate electrodes, the leads, and the instruments. Most of the problems will be caused by faulty leads, and in many cases you should be able to repair these yourself.

The instruments (e.g., diathermy forceps) are unlikely to give problems, provided that they are checked after each sterilization.

6. Ultrasound equipment

Ultrasound is used in medicine for both diagnostic and therapeutic procedures, but the equipment differs. For diagnosis, ultrasound echography is commonly used to produce cross-sectional images of the body. The Doppler technique is used mainly for blood flow measurement. For therapy, ultrasound is used in ophthalmology for lens treatment, as well as for lithotripsy of kidney stones and gallstones.

Modern ultrasound scanners are very reliable. They are also technologically sophisticated; the physician can only maintain the instrument as explained in the section on regular preventive maintenance (page 118). The hospital engineer should be able to rectify about 50% of all the common problems, as these tend to be fairly simple, and involve the transducer (probe) cable or power supply.

Physical principles

Ultrasound waves can pass through most body tissues. In the soft tissues, only longitudinal waves can propagate to any appreciable distance. Other modes (transversal, shear, etc.) are very strongly attenuated and can be ignored for all practical considerations, as regards image formation. The other modes of vibration can propagate in the bones, but cannot be used in echography. The main parameters of the ultrasound wave are its frequency (f), the propagation speed (c), the wavelength (l), pressure (P), and the intensity (energy per unit area per unit time, measured in W/m^2 or W/cm^2).

The relation of frequency (f) to wavelength (l) and propagation speed (c) is:

$$l = \frac{c}{f}$$

Body tissues can be considered to consist of particles, which oscillate about their equilibrium position when ultrasound passes through. Each tissue under investigation has a characteristic acoustic impedance, which equals the ratio of acoustic pressure to the particle velocity caused by the pressure, and a characteristic propagation speed, which is the same for all frequencies at the intensities used in echography. If the boundary between two media with different characteristic acoustic impedances is much larger than the wavelength, the incident wave is partly reflected while the rest is transmitted across the boundary and, in principle, refracted (Fig. 6.1).

Fig. 6.1. Geometry of reflectance and transmission of an ultrasound beam at an interface of two media with different densities.

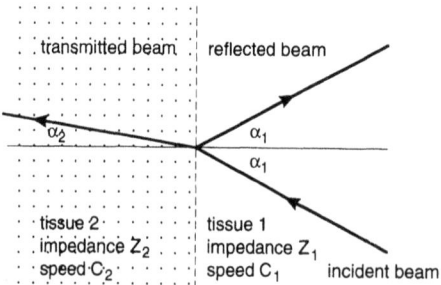

In the situation shown in Fig. 6.1, the amount of reflection depends on both the ratio of the characteristic acoustic impedances, and the propagation speeds in the respective media. The most important case is the case of normal (at 90°) incidence. In such a case, the ratio of the intensity of the reflected wave (I_r) to the intensity of the incident wave (I_i) is:

$$\frac{I_r}{I_i} = \frac{(Z_2 - Z_1)^2}{(Z_2 + Z_1)^2}$$

where Z_1 and Z_2 are the characteristic acoustic impedances of the first and the second medium, respectively.

The angle of refraction depends on the ratio of the propagation speeds: the larger the ratio, the larger the refraction.

The impedance of soft tissue is much lower than that of bone and much higher than that of gases. Relative values are approximately $1.5 \pm 10\%$ for soft tissues, 0.0004 for gases, and 7–8 for bones.

Ultrasound is attenuated by about two orders of magnitude more in bones and gases than in soft tissues. Attenuation is approximately proportional to the frequency in soft tissues, and to the square of the frequency in water.

The average propagation speed in the tissues is 1540 m/s, in body gases approximately 330 m/s, and in the bones almost 4000 m/s. Using the above equations, it can be seen that virtually all the ultrasound radiation will be reflected at a soft tissue/gas boundary, and that very little (about 6%) will be returned from behind bone. The angle of refraction at these boundaries is also high.

For these reasons it is not possible to examine the lungs, or the interior of bones, by ultrasound and there are many problems in examining the abdomen when there is a lot of gas in the bowel. Two-dimensional imaging of the brain is impaired by refraction at the bone/soft tissue boundary. The operator must be aware of potential artefacts in order to distinguish them from the symptoms of equipment breakdown. One particular phenomenon appears when the boundary between two media is wider than the wavelength of the ultrasound. Such boundaries act like a mirror and are called specular reflectors. The diaphragm, urinary bladder and gallbladder walls, blood vessel walls, connective tissue capsules, and ventricles are all specular reflectors.

An ultrasound scanner (echograph) transmits short (< 1 microsecond) ultrasound pulses into the body from a scanning probe, approximately 1000 times per second. Ultrasound pulses are reflected by different reflectors and scatterers in the body, and these echoes (reflected pulses) return to the probe, which serves as a receiver for the ultrasound. From the data, a two-dimensional map of the reflectors can be established. The relative positions of the reflectors are stored in a computer and displayed on a video monitor. Echoes of high intensity are shown as brighter dots on the screen. The image is of a section formed by scanning the body with the ultrasound beam. The echoes can be displayed in different ways (modes), as explained below.

The echoes along the beam may be shown in the form of peaks on the screen, allowing the distance between known structures in the body to be measured. This is called the "A" mode (Fig. 6.2). The "B" mode image shows the echoes as bright dots, with the brightness proportional to the strength of the echo. The B scan is obtained by moving the transducer along the body surface and displaying the B-mode images as a two-dimensional "map". In the "M" mode, the beam is aimed at a moving structure, and the system displays the changing depth of the reflectors. The M mode is often used in cardiology.

Fig. 6.2. Different ways of displaying ultrasound signals.

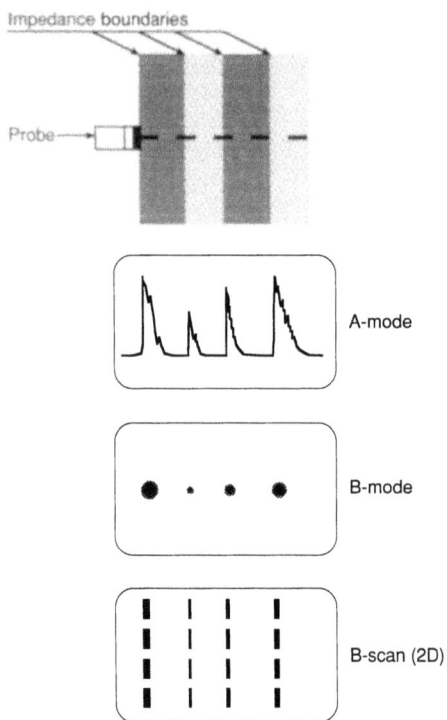

The scanner

Fig. 6.3 shows the various components of an ultrasound scanner.

The system consists of the scanning probe, the electronic scanning apparatus, and the video monitor. The scanner operates as follows: short, fast-rise-time pulses are generated in the pulse generator and taken to the scanning probe, which transforms them into short ultrasound pulses of central frequency determined by the probe resonant frequency. The frequencies used in general practice are between 3 and 8 MHz. The pulses are several cycles long. The probe contains one or more transducers which transmit and collect the ultrasound waves along a number of "lines-of-sight", by automatic movement of the beam in a section plane. The transmitted pulse crosses the body, and is reflected from media interfaces. The reflections return to the probe, where they are transformed into electrical signals. The ultrasound beam can be focused with fixed devices (lenses, mirrors) and by the use of phase-delays in composite probe transducer activation. The echo signals are

Fig. 6.3. Ultrasound scanner.

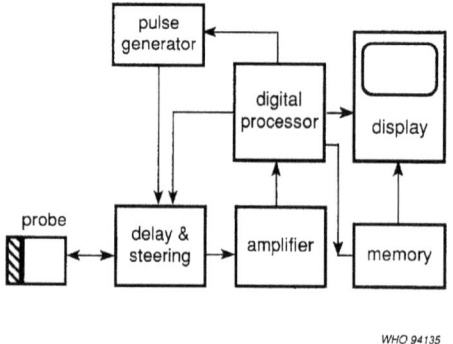

taken to the demodulator and a time-varying amplifier (the TGC—time-gain-compensation—amplifier) which compensates for the attenuation of the ultrasound signal in the body, by amplifying the echoes from deeper structures more than those coming from tissues near the surface. The amplifier has variable gain controls for echoes from different depths. The smallest number of TGC controls is three, i.e., the "near gain", the "far gain", and the slope (of the difference between the near and far gain). Modern scanners have internal preset TGC curves so that the controls serve only for additional adjustment or modification. The signal from the TGC amplifier is digitized and then stored in the computer memory, from where it is taken to the video compression amplifier and the monitor.

Scanning probes

A scanner probe contains one or more piezoelectric transducers. Each transducer is focused to a particular depth and can be classified according to the transducer arrangement as a linear array probe, a sector probe, or a curvilinear (convex) probe.

A linear array probe (Fig. 6.4a) scans in a rectangular format and is used in obstetrics, and in scanning the breast and thyroid. The probe contains between 64 and 120 narrow transducers mounted side-by-side in a 5–10 cm long array. On the

Fig. 6.4. Scanning probes with different geometry.

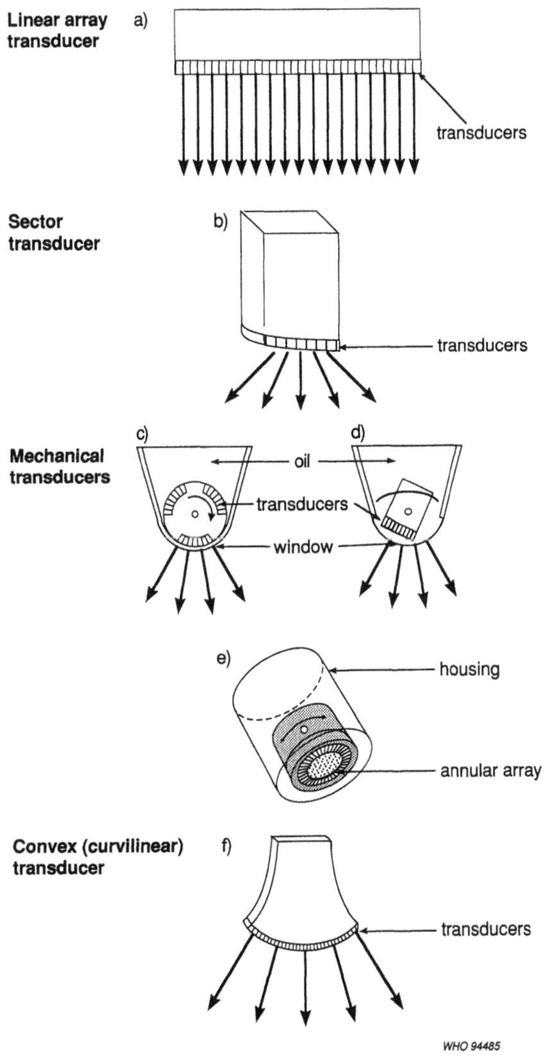

face of the transducers, there is a matching layer and an acoustic lens. Each of the transducers is separately connected to the electronic circuits, thus the connecting cable contains many thin cables, and is easily damaged.

A sector probe (Fig. 6.4b) "looks" into the body through a small acoustic window, forming a nearly triangular image. It is used mainly in the upper abdomen, and for gynaecological and cardiological scanning. A sector probe can be built with up to five transducers, which are moved mechanically with a motor for scanning (Fig. 6.4c and d). Alternatively, scanning can be achieved without mechanically moving parts by appropriately activating a very narrow array of transducers to achieve (phase-controlled) steering.

A sector probe may have an annular array transducer (Fig. 6.4e) which consists of multiple concentric transducer rings. If these are activated at different times, a circular focus can be achieved at any desired depth.

A convex probe (Fig. 6.4f) has an image format between the linear and the sector probes, and is useful for all parts of the body, except for echocardiography. It is built like a linear array, but the transducers are mounted on a curved surface.

The probe is connected to the scanner by an expensive, high-quality multiple cable. This cable is a common cause of malfunction.

Artefacts

Artefacts are those features in the image that do not conform to the real image for the part being examined. They cause confusion and often lead to incorrect diagnosis. Some examples are given below:

- A space filled with clear liquid appears as an echo-free area on the display screen. There is enhancement of echoes from behind such a space or cyst, while there may be shadows behind the edges of the cyst. This happens because the attenuation of ultrasound is much lower in clear liquid than in other tissues (e.g., the gallbladder has such characteristics).
- Intestinal gases obscure the structures behind them and can introduce multiple reflections (reverberation), which appear as uninterpretable echoes.
- Bones and calcified structures cast shadows on the structures behind them.
- Parallel structures can introduce reverberation (multiple reflections back and forth). This results in multiple parallel lines in the image.

The Doppler effect

If ultrasound waves of a given frequency are transmitted to a stationary reflector, the reflected waves are of the same frequency as those transmitted. If the reflector is moving towards the transmitter-receiver, the reflected frequency will be higher than the transmitted frequency; if it is moving away, the reflected frequency will be lower than the transmitted frequency. The difference between the transmitted and the received frequency is proportional to the speed with which the reflector moves relative to the transceiver. This effect is called the "Doppler effect", and the frequency difference the "Doppler shift". If the movement of the detector and the ultrasound beam are at an angle, only the component along the direction of the beam gives rise to the Doppler effect. This implies that there is no Doppler effect for plane waves at an angle of 90° to the direction of propagation.

At present, Doppler systems are used only in specialized departments, except for the simplest Doppler instruments, which can be used for the analysis of fetal heart beats. The latter can be easily used in any obstetrics clinic, provided the interpreter has been properly trained.

The general purpose ultrasound unit recommended by the World Health Organization does not have Doppler capabilities.

Recording

Ultrasound images can be recorded on photographic film, thermal paper, X-ray film, or video tape. Photographs from the video screen can be made with a standard 35-mm camera on ordinary black and white film. Such photographs are of good quality, but are not immediately available. Instant photography has the advantage of giving a print immediately. However, the film is expensive and a special camera and close-up lens are required.

Thermal printers give prints of a fair quality on special paper. The printer itself is relatively expensive, but the price per print is lower than with instant photography, if many images are recorded. Thermal prints tend to fade, if exposed to light, and in hot climates. X-ray printing equipment is expensive, but gives a high quality image. Processing facilities for X-ray film are required.

Video tape recorders are only useful in echocardiography. Digital or laser printers are expensive and only useful in large departments.

Maintenance and repair

The scanner has the following parts (see Fig. 6.3):

- probe (transducer),
- electronic processing block (amplifiers, TGC system, video amplifiers, digital data processors, digital memory),
- keyboard and other outside controls,
- monitor (display screen),
- power unit,
- hard-copy unit (printer or other recorder).

The probe is the most sensitive part of the scanner, in terms of malfunction. It consists of the transducer assembly, the cable, and a multi-pin fixable connector. The cable contains between 5 and 80 separate conductors.

The transducer assembly can be an electronically activated multi-transducer array (up to 120 transducers), or a mechanically driven transducer system (with up to 6 separate transducers).

Loss of part of the image or flickering

The most frequent malfunction occurs as a result of a break in one or more of the cable conductors. This may result in interruption of the rotation of the motor that moves the transducers, or cause intermittent rotation, flickering of the image, or drop-out of a part of the image. Such malfunctions are usually the result of mishandling of the cable[1] or of soaking it with gel. The cable can often be mended,

---

[1] It is important when scanning not to turn the probe always in the same direction, as this will cause the cable to knot and eventually break.

but if it is in a bad state, it should be replaced. The position of the break can often be detected by bending or gently pulling on the cable, while scanning, to see if this affects the image.

If the broken lead is close to the connector (which is less likely) it can be repaired by resoldering the conductors to the connector. If the breakage is close to the transducer, it can only be repaired by dismantling the probe housing, which should be done by a specialized service engineer. If the probe is dropped and the crystals break, any local repair will yield a probe of inferior quality. In such a case, a new probe must be purchased.

In composite probes (linear and convex), the failure of some transducers, or some of the cable conductors, can be detected by putting a pen or pencil on the face of the transducer and moving it from side to side. The reflection from the pen should not disappear in any position on the face of the probe.

Excess noise

The motor and the bearing in a mechanical probe can fail. Bearing failure is usually preceded by a prolonged period of noisy operation. Listen to the scanner during routine maintenance. In some mechanical probes, the bearing can easily be exchanged, but this requires care and should preferably be carried out by the manufacturer. If the motor fails, it usually requires replacement by the service engineer.

Gross image deterioration

The oil in the dome of the transducer must be air-free. The presence of air bubbles causes gross deterioration of the image quality. In some probes, the dome is transparent so that any air bubbles are visible. In the case of image deterioration (fuzzy images or moving defect in the image), first inspect the dome of the transducer for air bubbles. If air bubbles are detected, the oil must be replaced.[1] Although in some probes a good quality baby oil may be good enough, it is preferable to use the manufacturer's recommended oil. In well designed probes, refilling is a simple operation, possibly requiring the use of a syringe and a hypodermic needle.

In multiple-transducer mechanical probes, the transducers may have different sensitivities, or may not have been properly adjusted. This can be detected by putting a hypodermic needle obliquely into a beaker or glass filled with water, and scanning it with the probe. The needle image should not oscillate or change its intensity on the screen while being scanned.

Care of the probe

The face of the probe is usually an acoustic lens. It must be handled with care. Do not drop the probe, and avoid scratching the face with sharp objects.

Keep the probe assembly clean of oil and gel. Always clean the probe and cable with a tissue or damp cloth, after finishing work.

---

[1] Do not change, connect, or disconnect probes when the machine is running, especially if the image is not "frozen".

The electronics block

This part of the scanner is a complex electronic system located in the main box of the scanner. Because of its complexity, nonspecialized repair should be limited to changing a blown fuse, or repairing the high-tension circuit that supplies the pulse generator. Disconnect the scanner from the power supply before attempting any repair.

Change in image quality

A sudden drop in the sensitivity of the scanner can be a sign of preamplifier malfunction. A change in the grey-scale quality can be a sign of malfunctioning of the preprocessing unit, or a monitor problem. An inability to make measurements, or to change programmes, may be due to a digital processor breakdown. If only a part of the image is shown and the probe assembly is intact, it is most likely that the digital memory or the microprocessor is not working properly. Wavy movement of the image may be due to a power supply filter failure, or mains voltage fluctuations outside the working range.

When these faults occur proceed as follows:

1. Switch the unit off.
2. Measure the mains voltage; check that it is within the specified values (see below).
3. Check that the probe is firmly connected.
4. Switch the unit on.
5. Allow two minutes for warm-up.
6. Adjust the electronically generated grey wedge on the monitor screen, using the contrast and brightness controls.
7. Adjust all the controls to their middle positions.
8. Try to scan.

If the scanner still does not work, repeat the same procedure after 10 minutes. If the scanner still does not work, call the specialized service engineer, describing the symptoms of the malfunction.

If the scanner does not operate at all (the lights are not on, the fan cannot be heard), first check the mains voltage and the plug, then check the fuse at the rear of the scanner.

Mains voltage fluctuation

If the mains voltage varies beyond the specifications, repeat the voltage checks early in the morning or in mid-afternoon, when the voltage is likely to be the best available in the network. The scanner may operate properly when the voltage is correct. It may be necessary to acquire an appropriate voltage stabilizer from the manufacturer.

Recorded data

Specific hospital data (logo, preset adjustments, etc.) may have been entered in the scanner memory at the time of installation. Such data are retained, even when the scanner is switched off, because the unit has an internal battery. When the battery is exhausted, the scanner may lose some of the stored data. Replace the battery at the recommended intervals, before it is exhausted. Follow the instructions in the manual to avoid losing the memory during the change.

The following rules relate to use of the ultrasound scanner and should be followed by all users:

- Do not switch the scanner off and on in quick sequence. Leave an interval of 2 minutes or more before turning on again.
- Leave the machine running for at least 15 minutes.
- Always save the image after scanning.

Use the grey wedge on the screen to adjust the monitor, but if you need to change the grey scale during working, use the scanner dynamic controls, **not** the monitor controls.

Keyboard and front panel

All scanners have knobs and buttons that actuate potentiometers, which change the scanner settings. Some scanners have computer-style keyboards, and a few have touch-screen or light-pen controls. The measurement calipers are controlled by joy-sticks, trackball, or multiway buttons. Some scanners have slow digital processors; in such scanners, the computer may block if information is typed in too quickly. If this happens, switch the scanner off and restart after a pause of at least 2 minutes.

Controls

The controls are normally protected from the casual transfer of oil or gel from the operator's fingers, but may be damaged when liquid is spilled.[1] They will not stand rough handling. Even if used carefully, the potentiometers may respond intermittently after prolonged use, owing to poor electrical contact. Similarly, the trackball blocks may not operate smoothly, and will give a jittery response. Such problems can be temporarily alleviated by spraying the potentiometers with an anti-corrosive contact spray, but it is better to change the potentiometer. It is essential that the correct replacement part is used and checked after installation.

Power system

The power system for the equipment is installed inside the housing and is usually mounted at the rear of the scanner. During operation, this part of the scanner heats up; it is normally cooled by a fan. The power circuits can accommodate some variation of the mains voltage (usually $\pm 10\%$). The normal protection is a fuse (or two), located at the rear of the scanner, possibly under the cover. The power circuits are the first parts to suffer from surges on the mains network. The most common malfunction is a blown fuse, followed by a blown diode or thyristor. These can usually be repaired by the hospital engineer, provided spares are available.

The following precautions should always be observed:

- If the mains voltage is less stable than recommended by the manufacturer, a voltage stabilizer should be used.
- The fuses may be of a type that is not readily available. Spare fuses should therefore be obtained when the equipment is ordered.

---

[1] The keyboard and controls must be kept clean. Clean with a tissue or damp cloth after every working day. Do not spill any liquid over the controls. Do not hang anything on or from the controls. Turn them gently and smoothly.

- The ventilation holes in the scanner must not be covered with papers, forms, tissue, etc.
- The ventilator often has a dust filter. This must be changed every 3 or 6 months in dusty climates. If the original filter tissue is not available, a piece of double gauze can be used.

Monitor

The monitor is usually a commercial or domestic television monitor, and is seldom specific to the scanner. Other monitors can be used in parallel or instead of the original. This may not be easy if the manufacturer uses non-standard connectors, but a hospital electronics engineer should be able to change these. The scanner usually generates a grey or coloured wedge on the monitor, and this is used for adjustment. The monitor should be adjusted after the instrument has warmed up for a few minutes. Once the monitor has been adjusted for good visibility of the grey wedge, it should not be readjusted to change the ultrasound image. Further image adjustment should be made using the scanner controls.

The ventilation holes of the monitor should not be covered or clogged. Greasy fingerprints should be cleaned from the screen with soft tissue or a damp cloth.

Small or wavy image

If the image on the screen is smaller than normal, or if it is wavy or greyish and cannot be adjusted to its normal size, measure the mains voltage. The monitor cannot operate properly when the voltage is too low. On some monitors, the controls for horizontal and vertical synchronization are on the rear panel. If the image runs vertically, adjust the vertical synchronization; and if the image "collapses", try adjusting the horizontal synchronization.

The hard-copy unit

There are many different hard-copy units, e.g., a multiformat camera using X-ray films, instant camera, thermal paper printer, or a standard reflex camera. Each type requires different maintenance and supplies.

Acceptance tests

It is important that the whole unit operates well at the time of purchase. If it does not perform well, it is unlikely that it will work well at any later time. Carry out the following checks on receipt of the unit:

1. Inspect the packing crate and look for external damage that may have occurred while the unit was in transit.
2. Make sure that an operator's manual is supplied. A servicing manual is also essential for the hospital engineer.
3. Be present at the time of unpacking and installation. Check against the manuals to be sure that all accessory parts are present and not broken.
4. Make sure that the unit supplied matches the mains voltage available.
5. Carry out the initial tests when the mains voltage is at its worst, i.e., at a time of the day when the voltage is lowest and least stable. Do not forget that specifying your mains stability to the vendor is your responsibility.
6. Look for any damage on the probe face (the part that comes into contact with the patient) before using it.

7. Look for any traces of oil or contact gel on the cables, the probe, the keyboard and the front panel. When a new scanner is delivered, there should be no traces of oil anywhere on the scanner. When buying a used scanner, inspect the controls and transducer for evidence of oil or misuse.
8. If there is a phantom (i.e., a device with the same range of densities as body tissues, used for testing and calibrating ultrasound equipment), make photographs of several phantom scans. Write down the settings at which these were obtained and the resolution number, as measured with the phantom. Put them into a file for future reference.
9. Check all the probes by scanning your own liver. It should be possible to see the superior mesenteric artery. (This is a test of the resolution.) The dynamics of the grey-scale imaging can be tested by showing that the parenchyma of the kidney is slightly darker grey than the liver.
10. Check all the controls to ensure that they operate correctly and smoothly.
11. Check the electronic caliper system carefully. It must be possible to measure distances between two points on the screen. Check that the biometric tables are in the scanner memory, if they have been specified for the scanner.
12. Make sure that the presetting procedure for scanner settings is explained. Make notes in the operator's manual. These may be useful later if the memory battery fails.
13. Document the quality tests. Record your own superior mesenteric artery and liver/kidney; record a fetal head at 30 weeks of gestation with cavum septi pellucidi visible. Record all test images. Keep the records on file.

Preventive maintenance

The preventive maintenance that should be carried out by medical or technical staff can be summarized as follows:

- After each day's work clean the scanner, the probe, and the monitor with a tissue or a damp (not wet) cloth. Remove any oil or contact gel.
- Every 6 months (more often if necessary), clean the fan filter.
- Keep the ventilation holes open, do not cover with paper, even if the surface looks like a shelf. Do not put anything on any part of the scanner.
- Take care of the probe cable. Do not allow it to kink. Do not twist it always in the same direction.
- Do not switch the scanner on and off at short intervals; always wait for at least 15 minutes.
- If you are using a mechanical sector probe, listen to the noise from the probe. If it becomes excessive, call the service engineer to check the bearing.
- Save all the images whenever the instrument is apparently malfunctioning.
- Keep all the lids and covers on the scanner closed when not using the controls behind them. Switch the unit off and disconnect from the mains before opening any cover.

Routine testing

The scanner should be tested occasionally with a grey-scale phantom; if a phantom is not available, test by demonstrating that the cavum septi pellucidi can be seen in the head of a fetus at 30 weeks of gestation, or that veins of about 3 mm in diameter in the liver are seen at 45° to the ultrasound beam. A very good test of resolution is the ability to image the superior mesenteric artery in a normal adult. The superior mesenteric artery should be imaged transversally at the level of the pancreas, where it is seen as a roundish hollow structure. This test takes about 20 seconds to carry out, and should be repeated about once a month. If the scanner fails in this test, it must not be used in clinical practice; it should be repaired at the factory or by a specialized service engineer.

Necessary equipment

Ultrasound phantoms are commercially available for less than US$ 1000. One phantom is sufficient for many scanners, and the cost can therefore be shared among several institutions. Any large hospital or main health department should have an ultrasound phantom.

Specification of the scanner

A wide variety of scanners is available on the market. Therefore, before ordering, a specification must be agreed upon for an instrument that will allow the physician or sonographer to obtain useful and appropriate clinical data. The criteria must include price and quality. It is better to have no scanner than to have a scanner that does not provide useful data, since poor quality scans will lead to misdiagnosis.

Sector scanners are used for the upper abdomen, as well as in gynaecological and cardiological examinations. Linear scanners are used in obstetrics, and for scanning the breast and thyroid. A combined linear and sector scanner can cover all areas; convex scanners are also useful in the majority of body areas. A good generally applicable compromise frequency is 3.5 MHz, while 5 MHz is useful for scanning children and superficial organs. The original specifications for a general purpose ultrasound scanner were defined in 1984 by a WHO Scientific Group.[1] These have since been reviewed and updated.[2] Units of this type are now commercially available. Careful thought should be given before accepting any unit that does not meet these specifications even if it is less expensive.

The specifications for a general purpose ultrasound scanner are listed below.

1. The transducer design should be curvilinear (convex), or a combination of linear and sector.
2. The standard transducer should have a central frequency of 3.5 MHz, with accurate focusing. An optional transducer of 5 MHz is desirable if it can be afforded. The 3.5 MHz probe is a fair compromise between penetration and resolution, but the 5 MHz is very helpful in scanning children, thin adults and superficial organs. It is a worthwhile addition but should not replace the 3.5 MHz transducer.
3. The sector angle should be 40° or more and the linear array should be 5–8 cm long.
4. The controls should be simple and easy to use. Overall sensitivity (gain or transmitter power) and time-gain-compensation must be an integral part of the circuit. It should be possible to vary the time-gain-compensation from a preset level. However, this is not essential because if the time-gain-compensation is at the correct level for obstetrics, with a preset alternative for the upper abdomen, more than 80% of patients can be satisfactorily examined by varying the overall gain only.
5. The frame rate should be 15–30 Hz for the linear array and at least 5–10 Hz for the sector array.

---

[1] WHO Technical Report Series, No. 723, 1985 (*Future use of new imaging technologies in developing countries*: report of a WHO Scientific Group).
[2] Palmer PES, ed. *Manual of diagnostic ultrasound*. Geneva, World Health Organization (in press).

6. The frame freeze should have a density of $512 \times 512 \times 4$ bits (to provide 16 grey levels).
7. At least one pair of electronic omnidirectional calipers with quantitative readout is required.
8. It must be possible to add patient identification data (hospital number, date of the examination, etc.) to the screen and the final record.
9. It should be possible to obtain a permanent record (hard copy) of the scan. The hard copy unit must work satisfactorily in the same environment as the scanner.
10. There should be 2 or 3 imaging dynamics ranges available for post-processing. It is unnecessary to have a wider range of options.
11. The screen of the video monitor should measure at least $10 \text{ cm} \times 10 \text{ cm}$, preferably larger.
12. The equipment must be portable, so that an average adult can move it over at least 100 metres; if on wheels, these must be suitable for rough irregular surfaces, but a unit that can be moved without wheels is preferable.
13. The equipment must be suitable for the local climate, and be protected against dust, damp, extremes of temperature, tropical environments, etc. It should be possible to use the scanner continuously within a temperature range of $10-40\,°C$ and 90% relative humidity.
14. It must be possible to transport and store the unit safely under adverse conditions. It should not be affected by air transport or being moved across rough country in any vehicle. A specially designed case for transport may be necessary.
15. It is essential that the scanner can operate from the local power supply and is compatible with the voltage, frequency and stability of the local current. The equipment should be able to stabilize a voltage variation of $\pm 10\%$. If there is greater fluctuation in the local supply (and this should be tested before the unit is purchased), an additional voltage stabilizer should be obtained. These tests must be carried out before the scanner is accepted.
16. Many ultrasound scanners incorporate biometric tables in the microprocessor memory. These are useful, but care should be taken to ensure that measurements are made in exactly the same way as was used to provide the tables. Biometrics tables may not be universally applicable and should be adjusted for local conditions.
17. It is essential to ensure that servicing is available locally. No ultrasound unit should be purchased unless there are trained service engineers available in the vicinity. When in doubt, ask other local users of ultrasound equipment about the quality of the service and maintenance provided. This may well be the deciding factor when choosing between different scanners.
18. Service manuals and operating instructions should be provided at the time of purchase, especially if local servicing is not readily available.
19. Accessories for ultrasound-guided puncture or biopsy must be easy to sterilize.

7. X-ray diagnostic equipment

The production and use of X-rays

When a stream of electrons is accelerated by an electrical potential to a very high speed and then decelerated and absorbed by hitting a target material, X-rays are produced. Thus the main requirements for producing X-rays are:

- a source of electrons,
- a source of electrical potential,
- an appropriate target material.

X-rays are invisible. Because of their high energy and short wavelength they can penetrate almost all materials, but are absorbed to a different extent by different tissues. In the human body, absorption is high for bones, and low for muscles and other soft tissues. These differences in absorption can be shown on a photographic film as differences in density: the result is a radiograph. Thus, radiographic examination consists of irradiating a part of the patient with a uniform beam of X-rays and recording the emerging rays on a double emulsion film sandwiched between a pair of fluorescent screens. The screens convert the X-rays into light, which in turn exposes the X-ray film. The screens and the film are enclosed in a cassette for protection from daylight. After the exposure, the film must be processed, manually or automatically, in a darkroom by means of developer and fixer solutions.

X-ray examinations should be ordered only by physicians or experienced clinical health workers. "Routine" examinations are seldom indicated. A few of the more common indications and examinations that can be performed with diagnostic X-ray equipment are listed below (this is not a complete list).

- *Skeleton:* for fractures, and bone and joint diseases, e.g., arthritis, tumours.
- *Head:* for trauma and infections, e.g., sinusitis.
- *Chest:* for tuberculosis, pneumonia and other respiratory infections, heart disease, tumours, pleural diseases, and trauma.
- *Abdomen:* for trauma, intestinal obstruction, calculi, contrast urography, cholecystography, and problems in pregnancy, if ultrasound is not available.
- *Soft tissues:* for foreign bodies and calcifications, e.g., parasites.

Examinations with contrast media are recommended only when an experienced physician is available to carry out and interpret such examinations, and to treat the possible complications of contrast injections.

Components of the X-ray system

The components of an X-ray diagnostic system are:
- the X-ray tube, X-ray generator, tube stand (support), examination table (patient support), and control unit;
- accessories such as cassettes, intensifying screens, and film;
- darkroom equipment and other supplies for processing the exposed film;
- radiation protection devices.

X-ray tube

X-rays are produced in an X-ray tube. In all X-ray tubes, the source of electrons is a heated filament made of tungsten wire, the cathode. The area that is bombarded by the electrons is called the focal spot, and it is part of a metal body called the anode. The high voltage between the cathode and the anode sets the electrons in motion.

The anode and the cathode are sealed into a glass envelope, the tube, in a vacuum. This glass X-ray tube is enclosed in a casing made of aluminium, and lined with thin sheets of lead to prevent leakage of radiation. The tube is fixed in the casing at its anode end. The metal case protects the tube from mechanical shock, and also protects the users from radiation and electrical risks. The amount of protection has to be in accordance with international standards. The X-ray beam leaves the housing through a plastic-covered aperture called the tube port, or window.

X-ray generator

The purpose of an X-ray generator is to provide the high voltage that is applied to the X-ray tube for the production of X-rays. There are several types. One older type of generator, in common use in small X-ray departments, is the single-phase generator. In large hospitals, with a very good mains power supply, a more powerful three-phase generator may be installed. Recent developments indicate that, in the future, most X-ray generators will be frequency-converter, multipulse generators. These generators use a direct current (DC) source and convert the DC to alternating current (AC) with a higher frequency than the mains. These generators are much smaller, lighter and less expensive than conventional generators, and produce a high quality X-ray beam.

Usually, an X-ray generator has a number of fuses to safeguard the various circuits and their components. The fuses may be of different ratings and types, according to their use. They are usually mounted in the control unit, except in larger generators.

Tube stand (tube support, tube column)

The function of the tube stand is to support the X-ray tube so that it can be used with the X-ray beam in a horizontal or vertical position, or at an angle.

There are six basic kinds of tube support:

— integrated with the control unit and the transformer (e.g., a standard ward unit, or mobile unit, for use in hospitals);
— a column mounted on floor rails alone;
— a column mounted on floor rails, but also with a ceiling rail;
— a fixed column with a tube rotating around a central axis (e.g., a "C-arm", or a modified "C-arm" type, as used in the WHO Basic Radiological System);
— a column forming an integral part of the X-ray table;
— a carriage suspended from the ceiling, moving on rails.

With all these tube supports, except the "C-arm" or modified "C-arm", a separate vertical cassette holder, or chest stand, is needed for upright chest radiography.

Chest stand

The chest stand is a holder for cassettes that is used to examine patients in the erect position, for chest or other radiography. It must hold the size of cassette used for chest examinations, and be adjustable in height, strong and rigid. It may incorporate an anti-scatter grid (either fixed or movable) and should be able to hold cassettes either in front of the grid or behind it. With some types it is also possible to orient the cassette at an angle to the vertical.

Grid (anti-scatter grid)

When an X-ray beam passes through a patient, some of the X-rays continue in a straight line (the direct beam) and other X-rays are scattered in different directions. If the scattered X-rays reach the film, they will distort and spoil the image. The grid is a metal screen that absorbs almost all the scattered X-rays, i.e., those that did not pass through the patient in a straight line from the anode of the tube. The grid is properly called an "anti-scatter grid" or a "secondary radiation grid". The grid may be stationary or it may be incorporated in a "bucky" mechanism, which makes the grid move during the exposure and blurs out the image of grid lines.

All grids are delicate and very expensive: they are easily damaged, and are useless if bent. If not part of the equipment, they should be supplied either coated in plastic (for protection), or as an integral part of a cassette. Once damaged they cannot be repaired, but with proper care they will have a long life.

Examination (X-ray) table (patient support)

The examination table is used for X-ray examinations when the patient is lying down. It must be rigid, with a top permeable to X-rays, approximately 2.0 m × 0.65 m in size, and approximately 0.7 m from the floor. It must be able to support a patient weighing 110 kg without appreciable distortion. It should be impervious to fluids, resistant to scratching, and easy to clean. It may incorporate a "bucky" with a grid (see above). It may be fixed or mobile; if mobile, it must have good brakes.

Control unit

The control unit includes the meters, or digital indicators, that provide information on the state of the electricity supply, the chosen values of kV and mA·s (or mA and time), and the exposure switch. Often, the control unit is located outside the X-ray room. For busy X-ray rooms, this is recommended. If the control unit is located inside the X-ray room, a radio-opaque protection screen, large enough to protect a standing operator, should be an integral part of the control unit, or should surround it. There should be a lead glass window so that the patient can be watched during the examination.

Cassettes, intensifying screens, and films

Cassettes are the light-proof, rigid containers that enclose the X-ray film, to protect it from light. Within the cassette are two intensifying screens that fluoresce and produce visible light when irradiated by X-rays. The film is placed between the two intensifying screens, inside the cassette. The cassettes must be strong, rigid, and durable. They must provide firm pressure so that there is good contact between the film and the screens, but must be easy to open in the dark.

Darkroom equipment and supplies

A darkroom for the manual processing of X-ray films should have a master processing tank filled with water, in which two smaller tanks are supported to hold chemicals (developer and fixer). Running water is desirable, but alternatively the water can be changed frequently. If the workload is large enough, for example more than 15–20 patients per day, an automatic film processor may be needed. There must be a "dry" workbench, a film marker, safelights, and a thermometer. If manual processing is used, film-hangers and a timer-clock are also needed. If powdered chemicals are to be used, two auxiliary buckets for mixing, and mixing rods, will be required. Note, however, that powdered chemicals must never be mixed inside the darkroom.

Radiation protection devices

The essential radiation protection devices include a shielded control booth, outside the X-ray room, or a protective screen (large enough to protect a standing operator), with a lead equivalence of at least 0.5 mm, and with a lead glass window. There must also be leaded protective aprons, and leaded gloves, with lead equivalence of at least 0.25 mm, plus leaded rubber or leaded plastic strips with a lead equivalence of at least 0.5 mm, for use as gonadal shields.

Maintenance and repair in the X-ray department

X-ray equipment is complex and expensive: although minor maintenance can be done by hospital staff, routine servicing and repairs after a breakdown usually require trained personnel. Nevertheless, a regular routine of cleaning and checking will help to maintain efficiency and often provides early warning of developing faults.

Installation

Because X-ray equipment produces ionizing radiation and uses a high-voltage electric current, there are strict international and, usually, local rules governing all aspects of any X-ray department. These include specifications for room size, electricity supply, radiation exposure, and many other important details.

X-ray equipment should be installed only by trained X-ray engineers; even the transfer of used equipment from one site to another should be done only by trained staff. It may seem expensive, but incorrect installation may result in even more expenditure, and may be hazardous to hospital staff and patients.

Warranties and service contracts

The warranty given with all equipment must be carefully checked.

Service contracts should be part of the initial purchasing agreement. It is recommended that there be two routine, scheduled maintenance visits every year (at 6-month intervals) for at least 5 years from the date of installation. The first visit (at 6 months) should be without charge to the purchaser.

A written schedule of the maintenance required should be provided by the manufacturers, and each item should be completed, dated, and signed by the service engineer during each visit.

Log books

Log books are essential for proper maintenance. Quality control will be successful only if careful records are kept.

The front page should contain telephone numbers (and fax numbers, if available) of service personnel and suppliers or manufacturers for all the equipment, including films, chemicals, and accessories.

Every item, large and small, in the X-ray department should have a written record in the log book providing:

- the make, model number, and name of the equipment;
- specifications for the generator, tubes, and all other items, including accessories;
- date of installation (and by whom); total cost of the equipment and the installation (shown separately);
- address of supplier, manufacturer's agent, and local service engineer;
- a list of the technical service manuals provided;
- details of any variation or modification from the standard equipment.

Thereafter every service visit, fault, repair, change, spare parts supplied and their warranty, and any other event should be recorded and dated.

Similar records should be kept when items such as lead aprons are routinely tested, and concerning any other similar departmental maintenance (for example, the regular cleaning of intensifying screens, cassettes, etc.).

Tools for the X-ray department

Mechanic's tools:

- standard and cross-head screwdrivers, with insulated handles,
- coarse and fine insulated pliers,
- shift spanners and sockets (matched to the equipment),
- oil can, with light machine oil.

Quality assurance equipment:

- step wedge and spinning top,
- densitometer and sensitometer, if funds permit.

Spares:

- fuses for the main switches and electricity supply boxes,
- fuses for the X-ray room and darkroom lights and sockets,
- 15 and 25 watt bulbs for the darkroom,
- 40, 60, and 100 watt bulbs for the X-ray room, or fluorescent tubes and starters as appropriate,
- replacement tubes or bulbs for the X-ray film illuminators (viewing boxes).

Do not keep a spare X-ray tube at the hospital; it will deteriorate even when not used and the warranty will become invalid.

Daily maintenance schedule

X-ray room

Clean the floor, sweep, and wash or polish, if necessary.

Clean the X-ray table and controls. **Do not** use water on the X-ray equipment: use a dry cloth, adding spirits if marks must be removed.[1]

---

[1] It is very important to remove traces of contrast material and plaster from the table top (they may show on radiographs) and to clean off blood or other contaminants, but water cannot be used where there are electrical connections.

If the X-ray table is on wheels, move it away from the other equipment. It can then be cleaned with soap and water if necessary, provided there are no electrical connections.

Darkroom

Manual processing

Remove any films that have been left in the washing tank overnight. Wipe clean around the edges of the main tank. Make sure the washing water is clean and flows freely, and is at the correct level. Top up the developer and fixer from stock bottles.

Each morning and again each afternoon, measure the temperature of the developer, and adjust the processing time accordingly.

Replace all film hangers on their hooks. If any have been in the water overnight, wipe each one before hanging it above the dry bench.

If there is a separate film drier, remove all films and hangers. Check to make sure that no film has fallen to the bottom of the drier (remove any other material that may be there!).

If there are film carriers for wet films, empty the bottom tray, and clean the tray and the rack.

Automatic processor

Turn the electric power switch on and check the temperature after 10 minutes. Turn on the water and check the water pressure.

Check the levels of the developer and the fixer in the storage tanks. Some of the large automatic processors also have a washing agent; check this as well.

When the first films are processed, watch the indicators of chemical flow (usually near the delivery end of the processor) and check that the films are properly processed, washed, and dried. If there are clean, dry, but discarded films from previous work, feed one or two of them through the processor at the start of each day. This will ensure that the rollers are working well. Do no not use any bent, stiff, or distorted film.

Film testing

In busy departments it is important to run a test strip through the processor every day at the same time, for example at 10:00. Strip films can be purchased ready to use: alternatively, they can be manufactured in the darkroom. The best method is to expose areas of the film to a constant light source from a sensitometer and then develop the film. The test strip can also be made with an X-ray machine, but a generator of reproducible output must be used. In the latter case, to make a strip film, put a standard film in a 24 cm × 30 cm cassette (or larger). Position the cassette on the X-ray table, closing the collimator, or light beam, to the film size. Cover a strip 3 cm × 24 cm at one end of the cassette with a leaded rubber sheet. Put the step wedge on the other part of the cassette. Give the exposure normally used for a postero-anterior view of an adult wrist. Take the film out of the cassette in the darkroom, cut the film into strips so that each strip has a part of the covered section and also includes each step of the step wedge. Regardless of the method used to obtain the test strips, take one strip and feed it through the processor; it may be necessary to fasten the strip to a large-size discarded film to ensure that it moves through the processor smoothly. Store the other strips in a light-proof box in the darkroom. Repeat the processing of one strip of film every day at the same time. Compare the processed strip films against a viewing box; they should be identical if the processor is working properly. The covered section of the film should be quite clear, proving that the film was not fogged before the X-ray exposure. If there is a densitometer, read the values for density, at each step, on both films. This is more accurate than visual comparison. On a daily basis, it is only necessary to read three steps; the base and fog (lightest), and those corresponding approximately to optical densities 1.0 and 2.0. It is important to record the results, and useful to plot the results and to indicate on a graph the tolerances accepted.

Dry bench

Every morning wipe the dry bench with a clean cloth, remove any dust and pieces of film or paper. Dispose of any film wrapping paper, empty film boxes, name-marking strips, request forms, etc. Leave the dry bench clear of all unwanted items.

Remove from the darkroom any white coats, plates, cups, books, or other items that should not be in the darkroom at any time! Put them in their proper place.

Mobile X-ray unit or ward unit

Remove any dirt or dried liquids that may have splashed on to the mobile X-ray unit (e.g., in the operating room or emergency room) but **do not** use water. Use a dry cloth, adding spirit if necessary, but make sure that no liquid runs into the gaps around the control knobs or the edges of the meters.

If the unit is battery-powered, check the battery meter, or other indicator, on the control unit to make sure that the batteries are fully charged.

If the electrical connecting plug, or socket, gets hot after an exposure has been made, or during battery recharging, make sure the wires connecting the cable to the plug are not loose. Only do this when the plug is **not** in the socket.

Recharge the unit every night by connecting it to the power outlet; leave it connected during the day also, when not in use.

Office

File any returned X-ray films. If there are written reports, file them with the films, or send them to the records department as required. Complete the register with details of any late examinations from the previous day or night. Make up envelopes, and file any films taken the previous day that have not yet been properly organized. File the request form with the films.

Weekly maintenance schedule

On the first working day of each week, the following items should be checked.

X-ray room

Check that the equipment for use in case of fire is in the correct place. There should be:

– one fire extinguisher for electrical fires (water must not be used).
– sand in a bucket, or in sand bags.

Replace any supplies that have been used, e.g., cotton wool, sterile dressings, bandages. Check the contents of the emergency drug cupboard. Check that there are sufficient contrast drugs (for urography and cholecystography) and the necessary sterile syringes, needles, and skin cleaner. If the department undertakes fluoroscopy, check the supply of barium and all other items for gastrointestinal studies (enema tubing, cups/mugs, etc.). Order the replacement stores, as necessary, from the central store or pharmacy.

> **Instructions for cardiopulmonary resuscitation
> and for dealing with reactions to contrast drugs
> should be fixed on the wall of the X-ray room — always**

Darkroom

Manual processing

In addition to the daily tasks (page 126), check the film boxes and add new boxes of films from the store, if necessary.

Automatic processor

Lift the lid of the processing compartment, and lift out the developing racks. Wash the racks in clean water. Wipe and replace them. Be careful not to spill chemicals on the floor or elsewhere; damage may result.

Lift out the fixer racks. Wash them in clean water. Wipe and replace them.

Wipe up any liquid (water or chemicals) that has been spilt on the floor or the outside of the processor.

Monthly maintenance schedule

On the first working day of each month, the following maintenance should be carried out.

X-ray room

Perform the daily and weekly tasks, as applicable.

If the tube column runs on rails, clean the rails and the wheels of the column. Remove all dirt, fluff, etc.

Darkroom

Manual processing

The processing chemicals must be changed at least each month. Whenever the chemicals are changed, the tanks must be thoroughly cleaned.

Switch off any heating or cooling system and stop the running water. Empty all the tanks. Wash and scrub all the tanks, including the master tank, with a brush and running water. Mix new developer and fixer solutions. Use different rods for mixing the developer and the fixer. The developer is an alkaline solution, while fixer is acid. Do not allow even a few drops of the chemicals to get into the wrong tank or container.

Refill the chemical tanks with the new solutions: the developer must always be in the same developing tank, and the fixer in the same fixer tank as before. Never interchange tanks. Refill the master tank with water.

Automatic processor

Turn off the water and the electricity supply. Clean the racks as on the weekly schedule. Clean the developer and fixer tanks (using separate brushes for each tank). Refill with fresh chemicals following the manufacturer's instructions. Turn on the processor and the water supply.

Silver recovery

With either manual or automatic processing, collect fixer or silver, according to the manufacturer's or recovery company's instructions. If the fixer is to be transported to a central depot, it should be put into airtight containers.

Office

Add up the monthly totals of all entries in the patient register. For example, the total number of patients radiographed, the number of adults, the number of children, the number of chest radiographs, skeletal radiographs, etc., during the preceding month. Also, determine the total number of examinations.

Calculate the total number of X-ray films of each size used during the preceding month and check the stock of unused film, film envelopes, and chemicals. Order stocks as necessary.

Six-month maintenance schedule

Every six months, in addition to all previous routine maintenance, the following maintenance should be carried out.

X-ray room

Check all the moving parts on the equipment, particularly the brakes on the tube column and on the mobile patient support. If the brakes are mechanical, clean where possible. If the brakes are electric, and not working properly, request service. Do not continue to use equipment with poorly functioning brakes, since patients or staff may be hurt. Check all floor rails, wheels on examination table, etc., and clean as necessary.

Collimator alignment

Check the collimator alignment. If the collimator does not have a light beam, centre the tube on the middle of a 24 × 30 cm cassette, accurately placed in, or on, the cassette holder. Set the diaphragm for one size smaller (for example 18 × 24 cm). Make an exposure equal to that for a postero-anterior view of an adult hand. Develop the film and examine it on a viewing box. The square defined by the collimator should be clear cut and exactly the same distance inside the edge of the film all around. If the alignment is not exact, check to see if the tube casing has rotated, or if the collimator is loose. Tighten screws if necessary. (See below for tube rotation.)

Repeat the procedure with a horizontal X-ray beam in the position used for a chest radiograph of an erect patient.

If there is a light-beam collimator, choose the same size cassette, 24 × 30 cm. Centre the cassette exactly in, or on, the cassette holder, centre the tube on the cassette, and narrow the illuminated area by about 2 cm all around the inside of the edges of the cassette. Then expose and process the film as above. Take another cassette of the same size and repeat the procedure with a horizontal X-ray beam, and with the cassette holder in the position used for a chest radiograph of an erect patient.

Incorrect collimation

Misalignment will be shown by the exposed area being closer to one edge of the film than the other. There are two common causes. The tube housing may have rotated, or the collimator may be loose. Most tubes are held in place by two circular bands, which can be loosened or tightened by screws. Collimators are fastened to an X-ray tube on a base plate, often with four screws. These can become loose. Alignment of either the tube or the collimator can be more difficult than it sounds. Repeated check films may be necessary, particularly when there is no light beam collimator.

If the alignment is only slightly out, it is probably better to check that the screws are tight and then make no adjustment. If the alignment is badly out and cannot be corrected easily, notify the service engineer.

X-ray room and X-ray generator

Check the generator output. If there is a step-wedge, use it to make exposures at 55, 90, and 120 kV, with a constant mA·s, but varying mA and time. For each value of mA·s, the densities should be similar at each level on films developed in the same way, in the same chemicals, at the same time.

If there is no step-wedge, use any partially radiation-translucent object, for example, several ball point pens with metal covers. Expose the film, using different exposure factors, and process as described above. Visual comparison will show any marked discrepancies.

Check the timer. This can be done by using a metal spinning-top that has a small hole in the disc. The top is placed on a 24 × 30 cm cassette and centred under the X-ray tube. The cassette is shielded with leaded rubber so that only 1/4 of it is exposed. Twist the top so that it is spinning quite fast, and make an exposure at 55 kV, 100 mA, 0.1 sec. Repeat this procedure on each quarter of the film. The images should all show the same number of dots. For a single-phase X-ray unit, if the line frequency is 60 Hz, there should be 12 dots for each exposure. The number will vary with the design of the X-ray generator, but should be the same for each exposure with the same machine.

This is a very simple test, and not very accurate for complex 3-phase units. However, it does give a reasonable guide, and if there are discrepancies the service engineer should be notified. It cannot be used for frequency-converter multipulse generators, but these should remain accurate.

Darkroom

All the intensifying screens should be cleaned at least every 6 months. If the department is busy, clean them every 3 months.

First, clean and dry your hands. Then, in the darkroom, using the safe-light without any white lights, open all cassettes, remove the films and replace them in lightproof film boxes, with the matching sizes of unused films. Put the lids on the boxes. Turn on the white light, or take the cassettes into the X-ray room, open them and dust the inside carefully with a light, soft brush. Then carefully clean the screens, using warm clean water, cotton wool, and good quality soap or washing solution. (Do not use the sort of detergent recommended for washing clothes or saucepans.) Do not use too much water; use a damp pad of cotton wool with a very small amount of soap. Remove any soap residue, using another cotton wool pad. Dry with yet another cotton wool pad. Then leave the cassette open in a dust-free, darkened room (e.g., the darkroom) for several hours.

Never let water or soap flow over the edges of the screens. This will damage both the screen and the felt pad underneath it.

Check the screen–film contact. This can be done without any special equipment by carefully checking the definition of the lungs (especially the small blood vessels in the lungs) on a good quality chest radiograph. All areas should be equally well defined. Smaller cassettes can be checked by looking at the clarity and definition of any image, comparing the centre with the edges.

A standard, commercially available, thin metal grid that has been precisely perforated with small, well-defined holes is a better way to check screen–film contact. This is placed in front of a cassette, and the film is exposed, using an exposure equal to that for a postero-anterior view of an adult hand. The small holes should all be well defined on the processed film and the overall density should be the same. If it is impossible to obtain such a thin metal grid, a wire mesh screen could be used instead.

Uneven definition, or uneven density, can be due to poor contact between the screens and the film. Underneath the back screen, there are felt pads and these may be worn or flattened by long use. Alternatively, the cassette may be damaged and warped, or not fastening properly.

Inspect the cassette first. Check that the hinges are intact and that the cassette opens and closes smoothly. Check that the edges are exactly aligned. Check that the locks for the cassette are all working properly. If there are spring pressure straps, check that they are symmetrical and engaging properly.

If the cassette is satisfactory, the lack of pressure is probably due to the felt pads inside the cassette, behind the back screen. Alternatively, the screens themselves may be loose.

Screens must be fastened by double-sided adhesive tape. Ordinary adhesive tape or glue will damage the screen. When replacing the screens or pads, fasten the front screen (which will be clearly marked "front screen") by first putting double-sided tape all around the inside of the front of the cassette. The front of the cassette is the smooth, sunken side, without any outside attachments. Put the front screen into the well of the cassette, with the emulsion side upwards. Put the back screen on top of it, with the fronts of the screen surfaces in contact. Fasten the adhesive tape all around the border of the back of the screen and put similar double-sided adhesive tape around the inside border of the cassette. Put the new felt pad (plastic pads are not satisfactory) exactly in position on the back of the cassette and close the cassette. Fasten, and leave closed for 24 hours without film.

Care of screens

It is important to know the following:

- Screens deteriorate when exposed to light. Keep cassettes closed.

- Screens deteriorate with normal use over 3–5 years.
- Screens are easily scratched. Never touch the surface of the screen with your fingers, and always keep the screens clean.
- Liquid, especially chemicals and sweat, damages screens. Keep cassettes away from the processing tanks. Dry your hands before opening a cassette.
- To allow easy identification when screen marks appear on films, the back screen of each cassette should be marked by writing a small number in one corner, inside. Screen damage will show as a similar "shadow" on the same part of the finished films, for many different patients.
- All screens in a department should be replaced at the same time (because the X-ray exposure needed to produce the same quality of radiograph changes as the screens deteriorate).

Lead aprons and gloves

Each item should be numbered when new and recorded in the log book.

Every 6 months, each item of protective lead clothing must be tested for defects. Check by looking for cracks, tears, blisters, or other signs of wear. If there is a small tear, secure the edges with strong adhesive strapping. Then put the damaged area over a cassette and give a normal postero-anterior wrist exposure. Process the film, and look for a black line, which would indicate incomplete protection. Any damaged item that fails this test should be discarded (after a replacement has been acquired).

If fluoroscopy is available, each item can be tested using the fluoroscope; cracks will be seen immediately. This is a good way to test double-layered items, such as gloves; these should be rotated while being tested in this way.

Some types of lead apron have an outer plastic cover and the leaded rubber is not visible. These must be carefully palpated for irregularities and tested in the same way by X-raying any doubtful areas. Some lead gloves have removable leather covers, which must be taken off the inner glove before examination for damage.

Twelve-month maintenance schedule

X-ray room

Turn off the generator at the mains switch.

Visually check all the cables for cracks or irregularities, especially where a cable is bent. Check the cable–socket connections; make sure they are not loose or corroded.

Check the X-ray tube and the transformer (the other end of the cables from the X-ray tube) for signs of oil leakage.

Check the earthing cables (connected to the table, the tube stand rails, etc.) for looseness, damaged insulation, or any sign of wear.

These checks should, of course, be routinely made by the service engineer every 6 months, but it is also a good idea for the X-ray staff to make these visual checks at least every 12 months.

> **Be careful with X-ray equipment. It can be dangerous.**
>
> **Do not open the side or other panels on any part of the equipment. Only a service engineer will be able to correct any fault inside. If someone with authority insists on opening the panels, turn off the mains switch on the wall first.**

Before sending for the service engineer

If the films have varied in density—too light or too dark, or inconsistent

- Are the chemicals too old? Do they need changing?
- Have you checked the temperature of the chemicals, and are you developing the films accordingly?
- Are the films developed using a timing-clock? And for the correct time for each temperature?
- Are you using a different make of film?
- Are the screens in the cassettes of different speeds? (If so, label the outside of the cassette "Fast", "Slow" or "Medium".)
- Are the screens inserted in the cassette the correct way round? The front screen should be on the side which will be nearest to the patient.
- Are the screens fixed properly? The film must lie between the screens.
- If there is an automatic processor, is the unit running smoothly? Are the chemicals fresh? Is the temperature correct?

If the films are "grey" or fogged where they should be clear

- Is the bulb in the darkroom safelight more than 25 watts?
- Is the safelight filter damaged? Has it got too hot and changed colour? Are there any cracks, especially at the edges?
- Is the safelight too close to the dry bench in the darkroom?
- Are the films fresh? (Check the date on the box.)
- Have the films in the box been exposed to X-rays? Has the box of films, or a cassette, been in the X-ray room while patients were being radiographed?
- Is the temperature of the chemicals too high? Is the fixer too old?
- Is light leaking into the darkroom? (Stay in the darkroom with the door closed for 10 minutes and look around.)

If there are marks on all the films

Marks in the same place on films of the same size.

- Look at the outside of the front of the cassette. Is anything stuck to it? Have any liquids left a residue on it? (For example, barium, intravenous contrast medium, or iodine.)
- Open the cassette in the darkroom, take out the film and put it into a film box. Close the box. Turn on the white light. Check the screens, front and back, for

marks, scratches, or stains. Clean the screen if possible. If the mark cannot be removed, carefully draw a circle around it with a pencil or ball-point pen. This will show on the film, but the doctors will know that it is a film fault and not something wrong with the patient. Replace the screens as soon as possible.
- If there are no marks on the cassette or screens, and the film fault is a "dark" mark on the films after processing, check the box in which the unexposed films were delivered, or are kept. A small hole or crack in the box may allow light to mark the film. This is unlikely, but if there is no other explanation it should be considered.

If the mark on the film changes its position it is nearly always due to a small loose piece of paper inside the cassette.

> **Whenever faults appear on film and the cause is not found, keep the films to show to the service engineer.**

General rules

- There is no reason for anyone other than a trained X-ray service engineer to open the side or other panels of any item of X-ray equipment. If you are tempted to open any part of the X-ray equipment, resist. If required to open the equipment, turn off the mains electricity supply first—switch off both the switch on the control panel and the mains switch on the wall of the X-ray room.
- All moving parts of X-ray equipment should move smoothly, not stiffly or jerkily. Never force any item that does not move properly. When there is a problem with movement, check to see if there is any dirt or other obvious cause. Never force control knobs to turn. If a knob will not move easily, turn off the generator, wait 5 minutes, turn it on again and try once more. If unsuccessful, turn off the mains switch and send for the service engineer.
- The rotating anode tube makes a humming noise when it is turned on and is working. After an exposure the tube will go on running, gradually slowing down after a few minutes. If it stops suddenly, or if it makes a strange noise, or if the noise increases or sounds "rough", stop using the tube, and send for the service engineer. If the tube does not start rotating you cannot make an exposure at all. Send for the service engineer and warn him or her in advance that a new tube may be necessary.
- If any meter or light on the X-ray equipment does not work normally, contact the service engineer, tell him or her what is happening, and ask for advice. It may, or may not, be serious. Try not to use the equipment until you have consulted the service engineer.
- Water (or almost any liquid other than oil) and electricity must not be mixed. Keep water and other liquids well away from X-ray equipment.
- If any fuse blows and it can be easily replaced, use exactly the same type of fuse to replace it. Turn off the mains switch first. **Never** use a stronger fuse than the original one. If the same fuse blows soon after it has been replaced or repaired, or if other fuses blow quite soon after the first one, turn off the unit and send for the service engineer.
- Any unusual heat, smell of burning, smoke, or sparking is an indication to **turn off** the mains switch at once. Do not turn it on again until the service engineer is available.
- In case of **fire**, turn off the mains switch at once. Do not try to see what is burning or where the fault is. Do **not** turn the switch on again.

> **Do not put water or water spray on any electrical fire. Use sand or a specially designated fire extinguisher. If possible, turn off the mains switch first.**

If there is a fire brigade or other professional help in the vicinity, get someone to contact them. If there is increasing smoke or heat, leave the room at once, close the door and give the fire alarm.

Battery-powered generators

For battery-powered generators, see Annex 1, pages 143–144.

Selected further reading

Breyer B. Physics of medical ultrasound. In: Kurjak A, ed. *Handbook of ultrasound in obstetrics and gynecology*. Boca Raton, FL, CRC Press, 1989.

Hanson G, Holm T. Optimization of imaging services at the first referral level. In: *Congress souvenir book, 6th Asian Oceanian Congress of Radiology, 14–18 December 1991*, New Delhi, Indian Association of Radiology, 1991.

Health devices inspection and preventive maintenance. Plymouth Meeting, PA, Emergency Care Research Institute, 1990.

Holm T, Sandstrom S. Rational design of and specifications for general radiographic equipment. In: Chiesa A et al., ed. *Planning considerations in diagnostic imaging and radiation therapy*. Florence, Italy, Clas International SRL, 1988: 442–445.

Huys J. *Blood pressure measuring equipment. Principles, use, maintenance and repair*. Amsterdam, Tool Publications, 1992.

Marsh RW, Olivo CT. *Principles of refrigeration*. Albany, NY, Delmar Publishers, 1979.

Neureiter J, Tschenk A. *Technician's handbook for hospital engineering*. Nairobi, Acme Press, 1989.

Palmer PES. *Manual of darkroom technique*, Geneva, World Health Organization, 1985.

Waggfener RG et al., ed. *Handbook of medical physics*. Boca Raton, FL, CRC Press, 1982.

WHO. *Technical specifications for the X-ray apparatus to be used in a basic radiological system* (updated version of January 1985). Geneva, World Health Organization, 1985 (unpublished document RAD/85.1; available on request from Radiation Medicine, World Health Organization, 1211 Geneva 27, Switzerland).

WHO. *Guidelines for the installation of WHO Basic Radiological Systems (BRS)*. Geneva, World Health Organization, 1986 (WHO unpublished document, RAD/86.1; available on request from Radiation Medicine, World Health Organization, 1211 Geneva 27, Switzerland).

ANNEX 1
The WHO Basic Radiological System (WHO-BRS)

Scope

The rugged, high-quality X-ray equipment specified for the WHO Basic Radiological System (BRS) is ideally suited for small clinics, health stations, first-referral hospitals, and general practices under the supervision of a general practitioner. In these situations, the population served is often in the range 10 000–100 000. At this level, no fluoroscopy should be undertaken.

Clinical indications for radiographic examination with the WHO-BRS (partial list)

Skeleton: fractures, bone and joint infections.
Chest: Suspected tuberculosis, pneumonia and other respiratory infections, cardiac enlargement, tumours.
Abdomen: intestinal obstruction, calculi or other indications for intravenous urography or oral cholecystography.
Soft tissue: foreign bodies, calcification.

Intravenous contrast media examinations are only recommended when an experienced physician is available, and able to carry out and interpret such examinations.

The X-ray equipment and accessories

Specifications for the X-ray machine

The current WHO specifications for the BRS X-ray unit, with accessories, are summarized below. The complete specifications are given in a WHO unpublished document.[1]

The BRS X-ray equipment consists of a high-quality X-ray generator and an X-ray tube, together with a high-quality focused grid, and a unique tube stand, all of which are linked together in a sophisticated manner to produce an optimum X-ray system.

- The output of the generator must be sufficient to produce (*a*) a minimum exposure of 0.5 mR (5 μGy) in 1 second or less, at a focus–film distance of 140 cm, behind a water phantom of 30 cm thickness; and (*b*) 0.5 mR (5 μGy) in less than 50 ms at 140 cm behind a water phantom of 12 cm thickness.
- There should be a rotating anode X-ray tube, with a focal spot of less than 1 mm, capable of handling 20 kW during 0.1 s.
- The total permanent filtration of the tube must be equivalent to at least 2.5 mm of aluminium.
- The control panel should indicate the status of the electricity supply and the chosen values of kV and mAs, or anatomical thickness. Only four kV values are required: 120, 90, 70, and 55 kV. The minimum range of mAs values, all of which must be usable in the entire kV range, is 0.8–200 in 25 steps.

---

[1] *Technical specifications for the X-ray apparatus to be used in a basic radiological system.* Geneva, World Health Organization, 1985 (unpublished document RAD/85.1; available on request from Radiation Medicine, World Health Organization, 1211 Geneva 27, Switzerland).

- The design must ensure that the tube is always connected to the cassette holder in a rigid and stable manner, providing precise centring of the X-ray beam. A fixed focus–film distance of 140 cm must be used.
- A stationary, focused lead/aluminium grid with 40–50 lines per cm and a ratio of 10 : 1 must be incorporated.
- The tube must be provided with a collimator that allows restriction of the X-ray beam to the sizes of the films used (see below).
- The film sizes should be standardized, and not more than 4 sizes of film should be used. The cassette holder must accept at least the following three formats: 35.5 × 43 cm, 18 × 43 cm, and 24 × 30 cm. The addition of 18 × 24 cm is desirable.
- A movable pointer or other reliable system of centring the beam must be provided.
- The patient support must be rigid, with an X-ray permeable top, and it must be able to support a weight of 110 kg without appreciable distortion.
- Darkroom equipment must be provided with the X-ray equipment.
- A standard range of patient protection devices must be provided with the X-ray machine.
- The back wall of the cassette holder must incorporate a lead shield of at least 0.5 mm thickness.
- At least one protective apron and 1 pair of protective gloves, with lead equivalence of at least 0.25 mm must be provided.
- A protective screen, large enough to shield a standing operator, must be an integral part of the control panel, unless there is a similar permanent shield with equivalent radiation protection. The lead equivalence must be at least 0.5 mm. A leaded-glass window, no smaller than 30 × 30 cm, must be incorporated in the screen.

X-ray generator

The X-ray generator should use the frequency-converter principle. These generators convert a direct current (DC) source to alternating current (AC) at a higher frequency than the regular mains frequency (50–60 Hz). The higher frequency AC uses very small and often inexpensive components. The power source may consist of batteries or rectified AC mains.

Generators using batteries are preferred, as in many locations the mains supply is unreliable. Preference is given to lead–acid batteries, because the maintenance of nickel–cadmium batteries requires particular knowledge and skills, as well as expensive equipment (see page 144).

The exposure switch must be an integral part of the control panel, so that the operator must stand behind the protective screen during exposures.

X-ray tube and collimator

A movable mechanical pointer or other reliable system for centring the beam must be provided. The collimator design must prevent any part of a patient from being less than 30 cm from the X-ray tube focus. It should be designed so that it can easily be replaced by an adjustable light-beam collimator in countries where regulations make these mandatory.

Tube stand

A fixed focus–film distance, without angulation of the tube and the cassette holder, ensures the accurate direction of the primary beam so that the exposure of the patient and the staff is reduced.

Examination table

The examination table (patient support) should be easy to keep clean, impervious to fluids and resistant to scratching. There must be easily operated and reliable brakes on all wheels. The wheels must be large.

Cassette holder

The cassette holder, with its lead shielding of at least 0.5 mm, serves as a primary beam absorber and greatly reduces the need for shielding in the walls of the room. With a vertical beam, and without the regular examination table in place, it also makes an excellent small examination table for infants and for the wrists, hands, forearms, and feet of adult patients.

Premises and installation of the equipment

Two rooms, the X-ray room and the darkroom, are the minimum required. Three rooms are desirable: an examination room (X-ray room), a darkroom, and an office/viewing room. Storage space must be available, with room for a film file if the exposed X-ray films are to be filed in the X-ray department.

Fig. A1.1. BRS examination room.

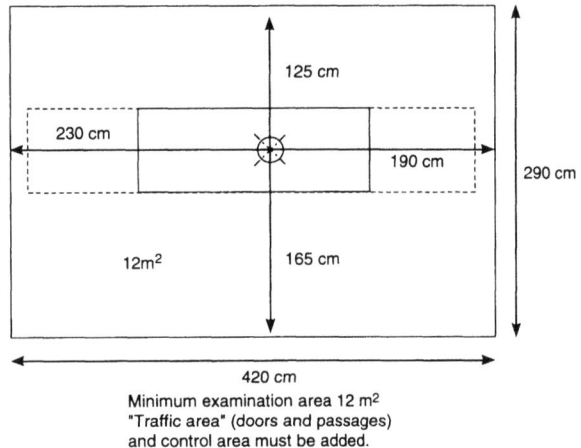

Minimum examination area 12 m²
"Traffic area" (doors and passages) and control area must be added.

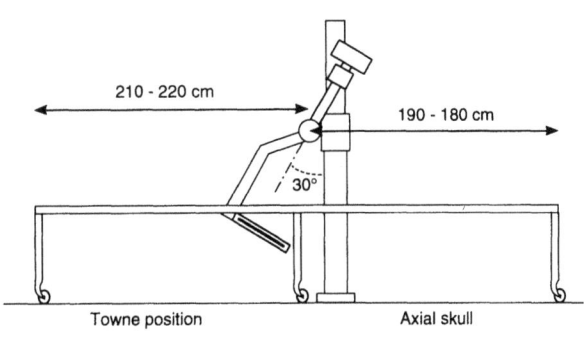

X-ray room

The minimum work area required for a BRS stand is shown in Fig. A1.1 and three possible floor plans are shown in Fig. A1.2. Additional information is provided in a WHO unpublished document.[1]

Fig. A1.2. Three typical BRS floor plans.

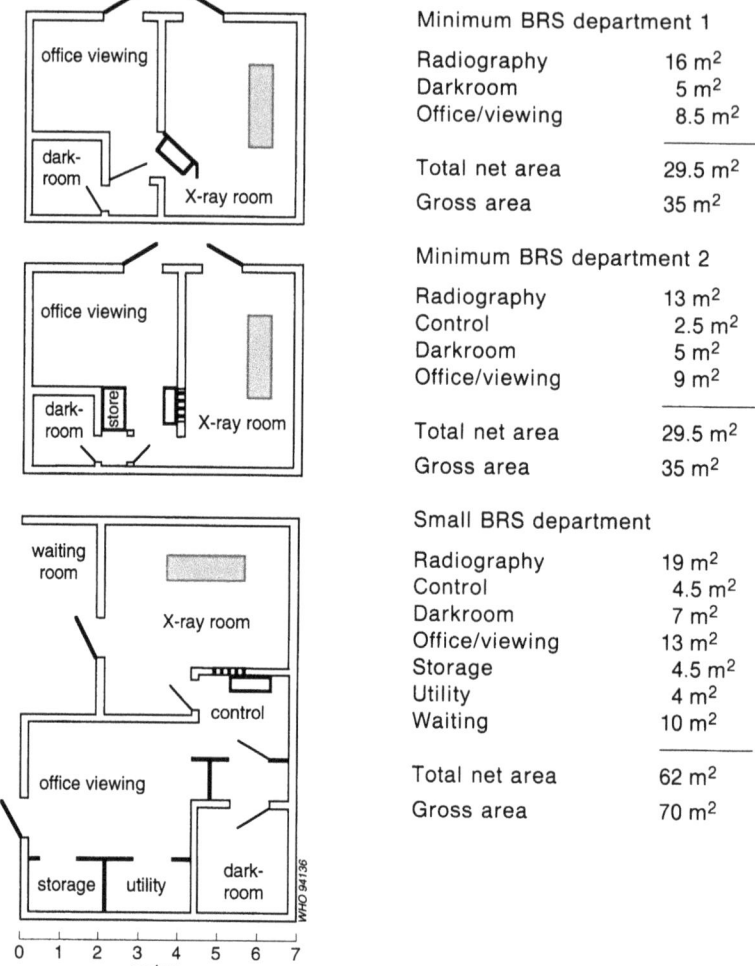

Minimum BRS department 1

Radiography	16 m²
Darkroom	5 m²
Office/viewing	8.5 m²
Total net area	29.5 m²
Gross area	35 m²

Minimum BRS department 2

Radiography	13 m²
Control	2.5 m²
Darkroom	5 m²
Office/viewing	9 m²
Total net area	29.5 m²
Gross area	35 m²

Small BRS department

Radiography	19 m²
Control	4.5 m²
Darkroom	7 m²
Office/viewing	13 m²
Storage	4.5 m²
Utility	4 m²
Waiting	10 m²
Total net area	62 m²
Gross area	70 m²

Darkroom

The darkroom should have a floor area of at least 5 m² when manual processing is used; no dimension of the room should be less than 2 m. If an automatic processor is used and the room is not continuously occupied, it may be as small as 1.5 × 2 m. A plan of the darkroom layout is shown in Fig. A1.3. Additional information is provided in the WHO unpublished document mentioned above.[1]

The darkroom must be entirely light-proof, even with the brightest sunlight outside. The light-tightness of doors, windows, and ventilation ducts must be tested carefully. No light from outside must be visible to anyone who has spent 10 minutes inside the room in total darkness.

---

[1] *Guidelines for the installation of WHO Basic Radiological Systems (BRS)*. Geneva, World Health Organization, 1986 (unpublished document RAD/86.1; available on request from Radiation Medicine, World Health Organization, 1211 Geneva 27, Switzerland).

Fig. A1.3. Plan of a darkroom.

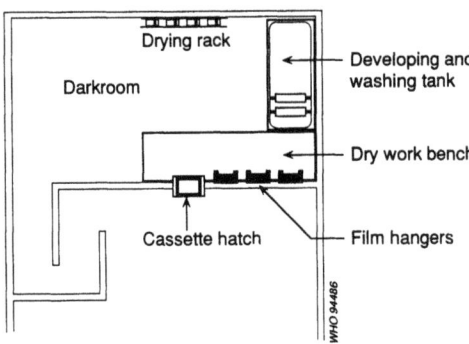

Three separate light sources are needed in the darkroom:

- General white light: a 40 watt incandescent bulb in the ceiling. (A fluorescent tube gives afterglow and is not acceptable.) The control switch must be **inside** the darkroom, 180 cm above the floor.
- Indirect filtered light: a 25–40 watt incandescent light directed upwards towards the ceiling, through a darkroom light-filter.
- Direct filtered light: a 15 watt incandescent light, with a darkroom light-filter, directed downwards toward the surface of the dry bench. The distance between the light bulb and the table surface must be at least 120 cm. This light fixture *must* have the words "max. 15 watt" written in large letters on the outside. The switches for the filtered lights should be located inside the darkroom at the normal distance above the floor for light switches in the department.

The correct safelight filters *must* be used: amber if blue-sensitive film is being used, and ruby red if green-sensitive film is being used.

If blue-sensitive film is used, the ceiling and walls should be painted with a semi-gloss, washable, chrome-yellow paint with no white pigment added. A pure chrome-yellow paint does not reflect any blue light, which might expose the X-ray film. If green-sensitive film is used, the ceiling and walls could be painted white, yellow, or another light colour.

Electricity supply

If the generator is to be connected to the mains, check the characteristics of the available power supply. Confirm with the expected supplier that the equipment is compatible with your power supply before ordering. Some generators may require as much as 150 A for up to 3 seconds from a 220 V source with a small impedance (0.5 ohm or less). Sometimes a 50 A slow fuse will then suffice. Generators using batteries or large capacitors may operate from a standard grounded 220 V or 110 V outlet, and do not require more than 3 A or 6 A during operation. If batteries are used, sealed lead–acid batteries are preferred, because they do not require maintenance.

If an automatic processor is used, the power consumption may be as much as 5 kW for short periods. Running water will also be necessary.

The electricity supply for room lighting and viewing boxes can be an ordinary earthed (grounded) wall outlet of 220 V, 10 A, or 110 V, 20 A.

Earthing

Earthing is absolutely necessary.

- Connect the generator to the main earth, if agreed by the electricity authorities; follow local regulations exactly.
- If not specified by local regulations, connect to an independent earth electrode close to the X-ray department.
- **Never** connect the X-ray generator to the water-piping system.

Installation

All X-ray equipment must be installed by the manufacturer or the local agent for warranty and safety reasons. It must be checked before acceptance. When equipment is being relocated, workers experienced in X-ray installation are essential. Incorrect installation may be both dangerous and expensive.

Operation

Personnel

The following personnel are needed: radiographer, assistant radiographer, or specially trained BRS operator.

The following special training manuals have been published by WHO:[1]

- *Manual of radiographic technique*
- *Manual of darkroom technique*
- *Manual of radiographic interpretation for general practitioners.*

Consumables

The following supplies are needed:

- X-ray cassettes and screens (all of the same speed and characteristics);
- films (all of the same speed and characteristics);
- chemicals for film processing;
- envelopes for films;
- record books for examinations.

Hazards

The operator and maintenance staff must be aware of the risks associated with the use of X-rays, and operate the X-ray equipment accordingly. This requires the operator:

- to use the correct X-ray exposure technique (kV and mAs);
- to adjust the collimator to the size of the film;
- to use protective devices for the patient when appropriate;
- to protect himself or herself behind the protective screen:
- to allow no one other than the patient in the X-ray room during the exposure (if the patient must be held or supported, a lead apron and gloves must be worn by all who do this);

---

[1] *Manual of radiographic technique.* Geneva, World Health Organization, 1986;
Manual of darkroom technique. Geneva, World Health Organization, 1985;
Manual of radiographic interpretation for general practitioners. Geneva, World Health Organization, 1985.

- to use the patient's family or friends when possible, rather than hospital staff, for holding the patient during exposure;
- to process the film according to the WHO-BRS *Manual of darkroom technique*, following especially the time and temperature guidelines.

Maintenance

Installation, service, and repair of X-ray equipment should only be carried out by specially trained and experienced service technicians or engineers. Nevertheless, some minor mechanical and electrical repairs, such as replacement of fuses or bulbs and cleaning and repair of brakes, may be undertaken by the hospital maintenance staff, provided they have received instruction from the supplier.

Spare parts

Do not purchase or store a spare X-ray tube. Tubes deteriorate in storage. As spare parts for equipment may be very expensive, they must be ordered only after careful consideration, and parts that may not be needed should not be purchased for storage. Because the supplier will be responsible for the major servicing, only those parts that can be replaced by the hospital staff—usually only fuses—should be stored in the hospital.

Special care

- Do not service the equipment unless the main electricity supply is turned off.
- Do not open the generator control console to attempt to make repairs.
- Never use a fuse of a different rating, or type, from that recommended by the manufacturer.
- If a fuse blows regularly, inform the service department or the manufacturer's representative.

Service contract

The original contract for the supply of WHO-BRS equipment should include the following:

- There should be an instruction book indicating which parts of the equipment require regular routine maintenance by the operator. This must be written in such a way that the reader does not need to be a skilled engineer to follow the instructions. Training for this routine maintenance should be given at the time of installation and during the period of instruction of all operators.
- There should be an instruction book indicating how to use the various controls, such as brake handles, etc., required for normal operation of the equipment. This may be part of the routine maintenance manual described above. All of these instructions must be compatible with the WHO-BRS *Manual of radiographic technique*.
- Copies of the WHO-BRS *Manual of radiographic technique, Manual of darkroom technique,* and *Manual of radiographic interpretation for general practitioners* should be provided by the supplier of the WHO-BRS equipment.
- Each item of electrical equipment must have a set of easily located test points so that the maintenance engineer can locate faults in the electrical circuits, on site.

Battery-powered X-ray generators

A battery pack may store enough power to give a life-threatening electric shock. Keep all metal tools away. Do not wear metal watches, watch-straps, bracelets, or necklaces.

Special advice for users of a battery-operated X-ray machine

If the quality of the X-ray films is not as high as expected, or the exposure has to be changed significantly to obtain good quality radiographs, it is often suggested that the batteries should be checked. However, this is seldom the cause of poor films because when the batteries are low the X-ray unit will not work. The commonest cause of a change in exposure and quality is failure of the processing chemicals. Before checking the batteries, make fresh chemicals, check the temperature of the solutions, and process a film for the correct time (see WHO's *Manual of darkroom technique*).

Read the manufacturer's instructions for battery maintenance.

In addition to the above, the following special instructions apply to WHO-BRS machines with battery power sources.

- If *unsealed* lead–acid batteries are used, the level of the water in the battery must be checked every month, and when necessary topped up to the proper level with distilled water. If distilled water is not available, the supplier should be consulted when the equipment is installed and the instructions followed; for example, freshly collected rainwater, without particulates or sediments, is similar to distilled water and can be used in most circumstances. A record should be kept of the performance of each battery, especially noting each time a battery requires water. The maintenance engineer should be informed if one battery requires more water replacement than others. Every three months, the acidity should be checked. Complete discharge of the battery may damage the cells, and such batteries will no longer be useful.
- If *sealed* lead–acid batteries are used, the BRS operator should check the indicator on the top of each battery at monthly intervals. If there is any evidence of failure, the maintenance engineer should be called. Sealed batteries should last for 5 years, provided they are properly recharged.
- If *nickel–cadmium* batteries are used, they must be fully discharged every 8–12 months, depending on the number of X-rays taken, so that they may be fully recharged. This is called recycling, and is a complex process. The supplier should be consulted when the unit is first installed to agree on the required recycling interval. Recycling cannot be carried out by the operators as special equipment and training are required, and it is usually better to replace the batteries with a spare set and send them to a central location for recycling. If properly maintained, nickel–cadmium batteries should have a working life of 5 years. It must be emphasized that recycling is a potentially dangerous procedure, because the batteries contain sufficient electrical power to cause second- and third-degree burns if not properly handled, and in some cases the electric shock could be fatal.

For all maintenance procedures, it is essential that the operators and the maintenance engineers are trained on the same type of equipment as they will encounter in the field. It is useless to train them on equipment from a different manufacturer, as there are so many variations. For example, some manufacturers provide an indicator to show whether the battery is high or low and in need of recharging. If this is part of the equipment, all operators should be taught to observe this regularly, and ensure that the batteries are recharged when necessary. However, other manufacturers provide automatic recharging, which occurs whenever the batteries are low, provided the X-ray machine is connected to the electricity supply. These batteries are therefore maintained at full charge, and will only fall to a low level if the X-ray unit is used many times when the main supply of electricity is cut off. These units also have a "state of the battery" indicator.

ANNEX 2
Set of tools, instruments and machinery for a maintenance unit in a district hospital

Description	Size	Quantity per individual			
		Technician	Electrician	Workshop	Store
Pliers					
Combination, insulated handle, chromium-plated	180 mm	1	1		
Half-round, insulated handle, chromium-plated	160 mm	1	1		
Side-cutting, insulated handle, chromium-plated	160 mm	1	1		
Multi-grip, chromium-plated	210 mm	1	1		
Circlips, internal, chromium-plated	8–25 mm			1	
Circlips, external, chromium-plated	10–25 mm			1	
Self-grip, nickel-plated	220 mm			1	
Revolving-head, punch plier, nickel-plated				1	
Pincers	160 mm		1		
Pincers	210 mm	1			
Pipe-wrench	370 mm			1	
Spanners, wrenches, and keys					
Open end, chrome-vanadium	4 × 4.5 mm	1	1		
Open end, chrome-vanadium	5 × 5.5 mm	1	1		
Set of open-end spanners, chrome-vanadium	6–22 mm	1	1		
Open end, chrome-vanadium	24 × 27 mm	1	2		
Open end, chrome-vanadium	30 × 32 mm			1	
Socket sets in metal box, 1/4", square drive	4–12 mm	1	1		
Socket sets in metal box, 1/2", square drive	10–32 mm			1	
Adjustable wrench, chrome-plated	4"		1		
Adjustable wrench, chrome-plated	8"	1			
Set of Allen keys on ring, nickel-plated	1.5–6 mm	1	1		
Set of Allen keys on ring, nickel-plated	1/16"–1/4"	1	1		
Allen key, nickel-plated	0.028"			1	
Allen key, nickel-plated	0.035"			1	
Allen key, nickel-plated	3/64"			1	
Screwdrivers					
Set of 4 screwdrivers, insulated handle, chromium-plated	M3, 4, 5, 6	1	1		
For cross-head screws	No. 1	1	1		
For cross-head screws	No. 2	1	1		
Watchmaker's, with 4 bits		1			
Voltage tester		1	1		
Ratchet		1	1		

Description	Size	Quantity per individual			
		Technician	Electrician	Workshop	Store
Hammers					
Sheet metal-worker's, with handle	200 g		1		
Sheet metal-worker's, with handle	300 g	1			
Sledge, double square	2 kg			1	
Punches, chisels, scissors, and awls					
Centre punch, chromium-plated	100 mm	1	1		
Set of 5 drifts	2–6 mm	1			
Cold chisel	20 × 150 mm			1	
Set of hollow-punches in metal box	10–50 mm			1	
Knife, pocket-type, chromium-plated		1	1		
Electrician's, scissors, nickel-plated	130 mm	1	1		
Scissors, normal, nickel-plated	200 mm			1	
Hand-shear for stainless steel, right cut	250 mm			1	
Awl	80 mm	1	1		
Tracing awl				1	
Measuring devices					
Measuring tape	2 mm	1	1		
Vernier caliper, stainless steel, medium quality	150 mm	1			
Spirit level	250 mm			1	
Plumb bob	200 g			1	
Mechanic's square, with stop	100 × 200 mm			1	
Files, bastard					
Flat	300 mm			1	1
Half-round	300 mm			1	1
Round	300 mm			1	1
Files, second cut					
Flat	250 mm	1			1
Half-round	250 mm	1	1		2
Round	250 mm	1	1		2
Set of 10 needle files	200 mm			1	
Rasp for wood, half-round	250 mm	1	1		
Rasp for wood, round	250 mm	1	1		
Handle for files	300 mm			3	2
Handle for files	250 mm	5	4		3
File brush				1	
Saws					
Hacksaw frame	300 mm	1			
Hacksaw frame	150 mm		1		
Hacksaw blades, for metal, medium	300 mm				12
Hacksaw blades, for metal	150 mm				12
Compass-saw for wood	300 mm			1	
Keyhole-saw for wood	270 mm			1	
Drill bits and threading tools					
Set of 12 drill bits in metal case, interval 0.5 mm, high stainless steel	1–10 mm	1	1		
Set of spare drill bits, 2.0, 2.5, 3.0, 3.5, 4.0, 4.5, 5.0, 5.5, 6.0 mm					5

ANNEX 2

Description	Size	Quantity per individual			
		Technician	Electrician	Workshop	Store
Drill bit	11.0 mm			1	
Drill bit	12.0 mm			1	
Drill bit	13.0 mm			1	
Set of thread taps and dier with wrenches in metal box M3, M4, M5, M6, M8, M10				1	
Set of spare thread taps, M3, M4, M5, M6					2
Set of 5 concrete drill bits	4, 5, 6, 8 mm	1	1		
Countersink bit, 8 mm shaft	90° angle			1	
Gimlet	5 mm		1		
Lubrication devices					
Oiler, with pressure pump	0.3 l	1		1	
Grease gun, high pressure	500 cm³			1	
Vices					
Hand-vice	150 mm	1		1	
Bench-vice	100 mm			1	
Joiner's clamp	300 mm			2	
Aluminium jaws for bench vice (pair)	100 mm			1	
Electrical devices					
Flashlight		1	1		
Hand-lamp, with extension cable		1		1	
Universal measuring instrument in case, digital reading, max AC: 600 V/15 A			1		
Soldering iron, 60 W				1	
Machines					
Electric, portable percussion drill	10 mm			1	
Bench drilling machine	13 mm			1	
Bench grinding machine	125 mm			1	
Protective goggles for grinding				1	
Miscellaneous					
Gas welding and cutting set				1	
Protective goggles for gas welding				1	
Acid tester for lead–acid batteries				1	
Tool box, 5 compartments, with padlock		1	1		
Flat brush	20 mm	2	1		
Steel hand-brush	3 raws	1		1	
Tweezers, straight	120 mm			1	
Spatulas	25 mm	1	1		

ANNEX 3
Basic laboratory equipment

The following basic equipment should be available in hospital laboratories at the district level:

autoclave
balances
blood-gas analyser
centrifuges (including haematocrit centrifuge)
flame photometer
hot-air oven
incubator
micropipettes
microscopes
mixing machines
pH meter
refrigerators
spectrophotometer/photometer/colorimeter
water-baths
water-still

This list covers the basic laboratory equipment for which there needs to be a service commitment, and does not include disposable supplies, i.e., plastics, glassware, etc.

ANNEX 4
Physical units

Relationship between °C and °F:

$$°C = \frac{5}{9}(°F - 32)$$

$$°F = \frac{9}{5}(°C) + 32$$

Absolute temperature K = °C + 273

Relationships between common units:

1 yard = 0.91 metres	1 metre = 1.1 yards
1 pint = 0.57 litres	1 litre = 1.76 pints
1 imperial gallon = 4.56 litres	1 litre = 0.22 imperial gallons
1 lb = 0.454 kilograms	1 kilogram = 2.2 lb
1 calorie = 4.2 joule	1 joule = 0.24 calorie
1 erg = 10^{-7} joule	1 joule = 10^7 erg
1 dyne = 10^{-5} newton	1 newton = 10^5 dyne
1 angstrom = 10^{-10} metres	1 metre = 10^{10} angstrom
1 atmosphere = 1 bar = 1 kg/cm² = 100 kPa	
1 lb/in² = 0.07 kg/cm²	1 kg/cm² = 14 lb/in²
1 mmHg = 0.13 kPa	1 kPa = 7.6 mmHg
1 lb/in² = 7.14 kPa	1 kPa = 0.14 lb/in²

Water hardness: 1 mmol/l = 9.6 French degrees (°F) = 5.4 German degrees (°dH).

ANNEX 5

Some common disinfectants, their dilutions for use, properties, and potential applications

	Dilution (g/litre)[a]	Contact time (min)	Inactivates						Important characteristics								Potential application			
			Lipid viruses	Broad-spectrum	Vegetative bacteria	Lipid viruses	Non-lipid viruses	Bacterial spores	Shelf-life[a] ≥ 1 week	Corrosive	Residue	Inactivated by organic matter	Skin irritant	Eye irritant	Respiratory irritant	Toxic	Work surfaces	Dirty glassware	Equipment and surface decontamination	Liquids to be discarded
Quaternary ammonium compounds	1–20	10	NE	+	+				+			+	+	+			+	+	+	
Phenolic compounds	10–50	10	NE	+	+	**			+	+	+		+	+			+	+	+	
Hypochlorites[b]	5–10	10	30	+	+	+	+		+	+	+	+	+	+	+		+	+	+	+
Iodoform[b]	0.075–16	10	30	+	+	+	+		+	+	+	+	+	+			+	+	+	
Ethanol	700–850	10	NE	+	+	**			+					+			+	+	+	
Isopropanol	700–850	10	NE	+	+	**			+					+			+	+	+	
Formaldehyde solution	2–80 (of gas)	10	30	+	+	+	+		+		+		+	+	+		+	+	+	
Glutaral	20	10	30	+	+	+	+		+		+		+	+			+	+	+	+

[a] Of the pure disinfectant, stored under appropriate conditions.
[b] Available halogen.
** Variable results with different viruses.
NE = Not effective.

ANNEX 6
Checklists for anaesthetic apparatus[1]

Draw-over anaesthetic apparatus

Keep a copy of this list by your anaesthetic apparatus.

Oxygen cylinder and flowmeter

Turn on supply of gas from cylinder, and check pressure and flow. Also check spare cylinder.

Oxygen reservoir

Check for proper assembly of T-piece, and make sure that air inlet is unobstructed.

Vaporizer

Check that the vaporizer is filled (using only stocks of anaesthetic in their original containers). Check that connections fit, and set dials to zero.

Self-inflating bag/bellows

Check connections and, if applicable, position of magnet on bellows.

Breathing and connecting hoses

Check connections and correct assembly of breathing system.

Breathing valve

Test the valve yourself and check it visually; the bobbin or valve leaflets should move during breathing.

Check for leaks

Squeeze the bag or bellows while using your hand to block the connector that joins the breathing valve to the patient. No air should escape.

Continuous-flow (Boyle's) anaesthetic apparatus

Oxygen supplies

For machines fitted with cylinder-only supply
Turn on the oxygen supply from the cylinder in use and check the pressure. Turn on the supply from the reserve cylinder, check the pressure, and turn it off again. Check that you have a third cylinder available to replace the cylinder in use when it is exhausted.

For machines fitted with a piped gas supply
Check the source of the piped gas supply. Check that there is a full cylinder of oxygen fitted to the machine in case the piped supply fails.

---

[1] From: Dobson MB. *Anaesthesia at the district hospital.* Geneva, World Health Organization, 1988.

All machines

Turn off all gas supplies except one oxygen cylinder or piped supply. Open all rotameters. Oxygen should flow through only one rotameter tube (the oxygen one!). If this does not happen, do not use the machine.

If the machine has an oxygen-failure warning device, test it as follows:

Turn on the gas supply from one oxygen cylinder (pipeline disconnected if fitted) and one nitrous oxide cylinder (if fitted).

Open rotameter taps to give a flow of oxygen (and nitrous oxide also if fitted) of 5 litres/min.

Turn off the oxygen supply at the cylinder. If a functioning warning device is fitted, an alarm should sound as the oxygen rotameter bobbin starts to fall (this may take a few seconds). On some machines, oxygen failure automatically cuts off the nitrous oxide supply also.

After the test remember to open the oxygen cylinder valve again.

Nitrous oxide

Check the pressure in the nitrous oxide cylinder in use and in the reserve cylinder. If the pressure in a nitrous oxide cylinder at room temperature is less than 5200 kPa (51 atmospheres, 750 p.s.i.), the cylinder is less than 15% full.

Rotameters

Inspect visually for cracks. Make sure that the bobbins do not stick in the tubes.

Emergency oxygen

Locate and turn on the emergency oxygen (bypass) button or tap. A high flow of oxygen should be delivered from the gas outlet. Note that this supply does not pass through the oxygen rotameter.

Vaporizers

Check that all vaporizers are firmly connected and filled with the correct anaesthetic agent (from stocks of anaesthetic in their original containers). Check that all filling ports are firmly closed, and that concentration dials are set to zero. A Boyle's bottle should have both the lever and the plunger pulled up.

Leaks

Check the machine once a month for leaks (or immediately, if a leak is suspected) by "painting" suspect areas with soapy water and watching for bubbles.

Breathing system

Check for correct assembly.

Index

"A" mode ultrasound 109, 110
Absorbance
  infinite 45
  light 44–45
Absorbers 94, 97–98
Accumulators (see also Batteries) 14
Acetylene 36–37
Alkaline batteries 14
Allen keys 145
Ammonia 52–53, 73
Anaesthetic equipment 70–100
  antistatic precautions 101–102
  Boyle's machines, see Anaesthetic machines, continuous-flow
  checklists 151–152
  draw-over apparatus, checklist 151
Anaesthetic gases (see also Vaporizers) 37
  precautions 37, 101–102
Anaesthetic machines, continuous-flow 74–78
  absorbers 94, 97–98
  checklist 151–152
  flowmeters see Flowmeters
  pressure regulators 94, 98–99
  rotameter tube 78
  testing 92–94
    procedure 93–94
    tools/materials required 92–93
  vaporizers see Vaporizers
Aneroid sphygmomanometers 63
Anti-scatter grid 123
Antistatic equipment/apparatus 101–102
  requirements 101–102
  testing 102
Artefacts, ultrasound images 112
Attenuation, ultrasound beam 109
Autoclaves 3–6
  inspection and cleaning 6
  non-jacketed 3, 4
  operating regimes 5
  steam-jacketed 3, 4
  use 6
Autopipettes 47–52
  maintenance and repair 49
  testing and calibration 50–52
Awls 146

"B" mode ultrasound 109, 110
Bacillus stearothermophilus (ATCC 1953) 6
Balances 8–13
  analytical 8
  beam 9, 12
  electromagnetic 8, 11
  equal-lever-arm (three-knife) 9, 10
  good working practice 11
  hazards/safety 12
  maintenance protocols 12–13
  mechanical 8, 9–10
  optical 8, 12, 13
  parallel-guidance 9, 10
  sliding-weight 9
  special tools/spares/requirements 12
  spring 9
  substitution 9–10
  unequal-lever-arm (two-knife) 9, 10
  unpacking, siting, installation 12
Basic laboratory equipment 148
Basic Radiological System (BRS) 137–144
  clinical indications 137
  consumables 142
  hazards 142–143
  maintenance 143–144
  operation 142–143
  personnel 142
  premises and installation 139–142
  scope 137
  X-ray equipment and accessories 137–139
Batteries 13–19
  alkaline 14
  carbon-zinc 14
  corroded 64
  dry 14
  lead-acid *see* Lead-acid batteries
  nickel-cadmium *see* Nickel-cadmium (Ni-Cd) batteries
  notes 19
  primary systems 13–14
  secondary systems 14
  ultrasound scanners 115
  X-ray generators 16, 143–144
Bellows
  Oxford 70–71
  Penlon 71
  self-inflating, checks 151
  testing 96–97
Blood-gas analysers (see also Electrodes) 27–29
Blood pressure machines see Sphygmomanometers
Bobbin, rotameter 78
Boyle's bottle 75
Boyle's ether vaporizer 91–92
Boyle's machines see Anaesthetic machines, continuous-flow
Breathing machines (see also Ventilators) 70–71
  checks 151, 152
  Magill 76
Bryce-Smith induction unit 78
"Bucky" mechanism 123
Buffer solutions, pH meters 27–28
Butane 33, 36

Cadmium lamps 41
Calibration factors, photometers 43
Capital costs 2
Carbon dioxide 33, 35–36
Carbon-zinc batteries 14
Cardiac monitors 67–69
  common faults 69
  earth-leakage current tester 68
  maintenance and safety checking 67–68
  spares 69
Cassettes 123
  chest stand 122

INDEX

Cassettes (*continued*)
  holders, Basic Radiological System 139
  maintenance 131
Cell counters 19–22
  impedance systems 19–21
  maintenance 21–22
  principle 19
  sources of error 21
Centrifugal force, relative 22, 23
Centrifuges 22–25
  analytical 22
  basic principles 22
  calibration 25
  good working practices 24
  haematocrit 22, 24, 25
  hazards/safety 24
  maintenance 25
  preparative 22, 24
  service 25
  tools/spares 24–25
  unpacking, siting, installation 23
Chest stand, X-ray 122
Chisels 146
Chlorofluorocarbons 52
Collimator
  alignment 129–130
  Basic Radiological System 138
  rotation 130
Colorimeters 41, 43, 44
Colour coding, gas cylinders 33, 37
Comparators 46
Contrast media 121, 128, 137
Control unit, X-ray 123
Costs
  capital 2
  running 2
Coxeter dry-bobbin flowmeter 78
"Cuvette error" 45
Cuvettes 41, 43–44
  good practice 46
  photometric measurement 45
Cylinders, gas *see* Gas cylinders

Darkroom
  Basic Radiological System 139, 140–141
  daily maintenance 126–127
  equipment and supplies 123–124
  monthly maintenance 128–129
  silver recovery 129
  six-monthly maintenance 130–132
  weekly maintenance 128
Defrosting 54
Deionized/demineralized water
  production system 56–58
  storage and handling 60
Desalination 59
Detector, photometers 44
Diagnostic equipment 61–69
Diathermy machines 37, 105–107
  bipolar 106
  hard-earthed output 106, 107
  isolated output 106
  maintenance 107
  monopolar 105–106
  radiofrequency earthed output 106–107
Dilutors 48, 49
Diode, light-emitting 41, 42
Disinfectants 150
Disinfection
  balances 11
  centrifuges 24
  infant incubators 72–73
Dispensers 48
  maintenance and repair 49
  testing and calibration 50–52
Distilled water
  production 58–59
  storage and handling 60
Doppler effect 112–113
Draw-over anaesthetic apparatus, checklist 151
Drill bits 146–147
Dry climates, care of microscopes 39
"Dry" workbench, darkroom 123, 127

Earth-leakage current tester 68
Earthing, X-ray generators 142
ECG machines *see* Electrocardiograph machines
Echographs *see* Ultrasound scanners
Electrical potential 25–26
Electrical safety checker 68
Electricity supply, Basic Radiological System 141
Electrocardiograph (ECG) machines 67–69
  common faults 69
  earth-leakage current tester 68
  maintenance and safety checking 67–68
  spares 69
Electrodes (*see also* pH meters) 25–29
  calomel (dimercury chloride) 27, 28
  characteristics 26–27
  glass 27, 28
  hazards 29
  ion-selective 27
  packing 29
  potential curve 27
  reference 25, 27, 28
  repairs 29
Electron microscopes 38
Entrainers
  Farman 74
  oxygen 73–74
Epstein-Macintosh-Oxford (EMO) vaporizer 74, 78, 85–91
  cleaning and sterilizing 87–88
  closing mechanism 87, 90–91
  fault-finding and rectification 88–91
  filling port 87
  level indicator 86
  safety release valve 87
  temperature compensating unit 87, 89–90
  water compartment 87
Ethanol 150
Ether 37
  Boyle's vaporizer 91–92
  Epstein-Macintosh-Oxford vaporizer 85, 88
Exchange resins, demineralizers 56, 57

Farman entrainer 74
Files
   bastard 146
   second cut 146
Films, X-ray *see* X-ray films
Filters
   darkroom 141
   flame photometers 30, 31
   photometers 43, 46
   water 59–60
Fire
   equipment, X-ray room 127
   operating room precautions 37, 101–102
   X-ray department 134–135
Flame emission photometry 29
Flame photometers 29-33
   calibration 33
   good working practice 31–32
   hazards 32
   maintenance 31, 32
   operation 31
   repair 33
   service 32
   services required 30
   tools/spares 32
   unpacking, siting, installation 30–31
Flow-control valves 75
Flow indicators 75–78
Flowmeters 75–77, 98–99
   after-service testing 77
   checks 151
   Coxeter dry-bobbin 78
   faults 77
   servicing 75–77
   testing 93, 99
Footwear, antistatic testing 102
Formaldehyde solution (formalin) 72–73, 150
Freezers (*see also* Refrigerators)
   installation 54
   maintenance 55
Fuses, X-ray generator 122, 134

Gas cylinders 33–37
   anaesthetic machines 75, 151, 152
   colour coding 33, 37
   hazardous gases 35–37
   maintenance 33–35
   reducing valves 34–35, 75
   safe use 33–35
Gas machines *see* Anaesthetic machines, continuous-flow
Gases 33–37
   anaesthetic *see* Anaesthetic gases
   flow indicators 75–78
   hazardous, special requirements for use 35–37
Glutaral 150
Gonadal shields, leaded 124
Grating, transmission 42
Grid, anti-scatter (secondary radiation) 123

Haematocrit centrifuges 22, 24, 25
Halothane 78
Hammers 146
Hardness, water 57

Holmium oxide glass filter 43
Hot-air ovens 6–7
Hot climates
   care of microscopes 39
   use of Ni-Cd batteries 17–18
Humid climates, care of microscopes 39
Humidity, antistatic effects 101
Hydrogen 35
Hydrogen ion concentration 27
Hypochlorites 150

Impedance
   acoustic 108–109
   cell counting 19–21
Incubators
   infant *see* Infant incubators
   laboratory 7
Infant incubators 71–73
   cleaning 72–73
   disinfection 72–73
   maintenance 72
Installation 1–2
   balances 12
   Basic Radiological System 142
   centrifuges 23
   flame photometers 30–31
   light microscopes 38
   pH meters 28
   photometers 46
   refrigerators and freezers 54
   X-ray equipment 124
Instruments, maintenance unit 145–147
Intensifying screens 123
   care 131–132
   cleaning 130–131
Iodoform 150
Ions, measurement 27, 29–30
Isopropanol 150

Keys, Allen 145

Laboratory equipment 3–60
   basic 148
Lambert-Beer law 41, 44
Laryngoscope 65–66
Lead-acid batteries 14–16
   recharging 16
   use 14–15
   X-ray generators 16, 144
Lead aprons/gloves 124, 132
Lead shields 124
Leukocyte counting 21
Light microscopes 38–41
Light sources
   darkroom 141
   photometers 42
Lithium (Li) 29, 30
Log books 124–125
Low-airway-pressure alarm 97
Low-oxygen alarm 97
Lubrification devices 147

M mode ultrasound 109
Machinery, maintenance unit 145–147
Magill breathing system 75

Maintenance unit, set of tools/instruments/ machinery 145–147
Manuals
 Basic Radiological System 142
 operating 3
Measuring devices 146
"Megger" 67, 68
Mercury 62
Mercury lamps 41, 42
Methanol 73
Microscopes 37–41
 cleaning 38–39
 electron 38
 hazards 40
 installation 38
 light 38–41
 maintenance 39–40
 precautions in hot climates 39
 repairs 40
 tools/spares 40–41
 use 39–40
Mobile X-ray units 127
Monitors, ultrasound scanners 117
Monochromators 41, 42–43
"Motor-boating" 77, 99
Muitiplier, photometers 44

Needle valves 75
Nernst equation 26
Nickel-cadmium (Ni-Cd) batteries 14, 16–19
 control of capacity 19
 gas-tight 17
 recharging 18
 recycling 144
 storage 18
 use at high ambient temperatures 17–18
 X-ray generators 144
Nitrogen 33, 36
Nitrous oxide 75, 94, 152
Nitrous oxide/oxygen mixtures 36

Office/viewing room, X-ray department
 Basic Radiological System 139, 140
 maintenance 127, 129
Operating table 102–103
Operation room equipment 101–107
Ophthalmoscope 64
 corroded batteries 64
 faulty on/off switch 64
 head 64
 rheostat 64
Otoscope 64–65
Ovens, hot-air 6–7
Oxford bellows 70–71
Oxford miniature vaporizer (OMV) 74, 79–85
 cleaning 79, 80–82
 pointer setting 83
 repairs 84
 servicing equipment 85
 testing for leaks 83
Oxygen 35, 37
 anaesthetic machine supply 75, 94, 151–152
 analysers 100
 cylinders, checks 151
 emergency 152
 entrainment systems 73–74
 reservoir 151
 therapy unit 98
Oxygen-failure warning whistle 93, 152
Oxygen-flush valve 93

Patient support (X-rays) *see* X-ray examination table
Peleus ball 49
Penlon bellows unit 71
Personnel 1
 Basic Radiological System 142
pH meters (*see also* Electrodes) 27–29
 good practice 28
 installation 28
Phantoms, ultrasound 118, 119
Phenolic compounds 150
Photographs, ultrasound images 113
Photometers 41–47
 comparators 46
 cuvettes 43–44
 detector and multiplier 44
 double-beam 41
 filters 43
 flame *see* Flame photometers
 good practice 46
 hazards 46
 light sources 42
 maintenance 47
 monochromators 42–43
 repair 47
 service 47
 single-beam 41
 tools/spares 47
 unpacking, siting, installation 46
 use 44–46
Pin-index system 75
Pipettes 47–52
 maintenance and repair 49
 mechanical 48
 Sanz 48
 testing and calibration 50–52
Pipetting 49–50
Piston suction pumps 104
Platelet counting 21
Pliers 145
Potassium (K) 29, 30
Potassium dichromate solution 43
Potentiometric chain 25
Premises, Basic Radiological System 139–142
Pressure gauges 75, 94
Pressure regulators *see* Reducing valves
Printers, ultrasound images 113
Prism 42
Probes, ultrasound (*see also* Transducers) 111–112, 113
 care 114
 malfunction 114
Propane 36
Punches 146
Purchasing 1–2

Quaternary ammonium compounds 150

Radiation protection devices 124, 138

Recharging
  lead-acid batteries 16
  Ni-Cd batteries 18
Recycling, Ni-Cd batteries 144
Red blood cell counting 21
Reducing valves (pressure regulators) 34–35, 75, 98–99
  setting output pressure 98–99
  testing 99
Reduction potentials, metals 13
Reference absorbing solution/material, photometers 43
Reference electrodes 25, 27, 28
Reflection, ultrasound beam 108–109
Refrigerators 52–56
  absorption-type 52–53, 55
  changing heating element 55–56
  compression-type 53–54, 55
  door gaskets 55
  good practice 54
  installation 54
  maintenance 54–56
    daily checks 54
    monthly checks 55
  spares/tools 56
Relative centrifugal force 22, 23
Resuscitation equipment 70–100
Rotameters 75, 78
  checks 152
Rubber, antistatic 101–102

Safety checker, electrical 68
"Salt error" 27
Sanz pipettes 48
Saws 146
Scissors 146
Screens, intensifying *see* Intensifying screens
Screwdrivers 145
Service contracts
  Basic Radiological System 143
  X-ray equipment 124
Silver recovery, darkroom 129
Sodium (Na) 29, 30
Solar-powered water still 59
Spanners 145
Spectrometers (*see also* Photometers) 41–47
  light source 42
  monochromators 43
  wavelength calibration 47
Specular reflectors 109
Speculum, otoscope 64–65
Sphygmomanometers (blood pressure machines) 61–64
  aneroid 63
  electronic 63–64
  mercury 61–63
Staff *see* Personnel
Steam sterilization 3–6
Step-wedge 130
Sterilization
  Epstein-Macintosh-Oxford vaporizer 87–88
  hot air 6–7
  steam 3–6
Stethoscopes 67

Storage
  deionized/distilled water 60
  gas cylinders 34
  lead-acid batteries 18
  X-ray films 139, 140
Suction machines 103–105
  electric 103, 104
  foot-operated 104, 105
  maintenance 105
  piston pumps 104
  repair 105
  wall-fitted 103–104
Sulfuric acid 14, 15

Table
  operating 102–103
  X-ray examination *see* X-ray examination table
Temperature
  electrode potential curve and 27
  high ambient *see* Hot climates
  hot air sterilization 7
  laboratory incubators 7
  steam sterilization 5
  units 149
  water-baths 7
Thermal prints, ultrasound images 113
Threading tools 146–147
Time-varying (TGC) amplifier 111
Timer, X-ray exposure 130
Tools, maintenance unit 145–147
Training 1
  Basic Radiological System 142
Transducers (*see also* Probes, ultrasound) 111–112, 113
  annular array 112
  convex (curvilinear) 111, 112
  linear array 111–112, 119
  malfunction 114
  mechanical 111, 112
  sector 111, 112, 119
Transmission, ultrasound beam 108–109
Trichloroethylene 37
Trolley castor tyres, antistatic testing 102
Tungsten-halogen lamps 41, 42

Ultrasound 108–120
  Doppler effect 112–113
  image 109
    artefacts 112
    change in quality 115
    display modes 109, 110
    gross deterioration 114
    loss of part/flickering 113–114
    recording 113
    small or wavy 117
  phantoms 118, 119
  physical principles 108–109
  probes *see* Probes, ultrasound
  transducers *see* Transducers
Ultrasound scanners 108, 109, 110–111
  acceptance tests 117–118
  cable 112
  malfunction 113–114

Ultrasound scanners (*continued*)
  controls 116
  electronics block 115
  excessive noise 114
  hard-copy unit 113, 117
  keyboard and front panel 116
  mains voltage fluctuation 115
  maintenance 113–119
  monitors 117
  power system 116–117
  preventive maintenance 118
  recorded data 115–116
  repair 113–119
  routine testing 118–119
  specifications 119–120
Units, physical 149

Valves
  breathing, checks 151
  flow-control (needle) 75
  oxygen-flush 93
  reducing *see* Reducing valves
  ventilator, testing 96, 97
Vaporizers (*see also* Epstein-Macintosh-Oxford (EMO) vaporizer; Oxford miniature vaporizer) 75, 79–85
  Boyle's ether 91–92
  checks 151, 152
  testing 94
Ventilators (*see also* Breathing machines)
  bellows 96–97
  controller 97
  testing 92, 94–97
    procedure 95–96
    tools/materials required 94
Vices 147
Video monitors, ultrasound scanners 117

Warranties, X-ray equipment 124
Water
  demineralization 56–58
  distillation 58–59
  filters 59–60
  hardness 57
  purification systems 56–60
Water-baths 7–8
  inspection and cleaning 8
  use 8
Water still 58
  simple solar-powered 59
WHO Basic Radiological System *see* Basic Radiological System
Wrenches 145

X-ray diagnostic equipment 121–135

Basic Radiological System 137–139
  components 121–124
  installation 124
  maintenance 124–133
    general rules 134–135
    log books 124–125
    schedules 127–132
    tools/spares 125
    warranties and service contracts 124
  repair 133–135
X-ray examination table (patient support) 123
  Basic Radiological System 139
  maintenance 125–126, 129
X-ray films 123
  automatic processor 123
    daily maintenance 126
    monthly maintenance 129
    weekly maintenance 128
  "grey" or fogged 133
  manual processing 123, 124
    daily maintenance 126
    monthly maintenance 128–129
    weekly maintenance 128
  marks on 133–134
  tests 126–127
  variations in intensity 133
X-ray generators 122
  Basic Radiological System 138, 141, 142
  battery-powered 16, 143–144
  six-monthly maintenance 130
X-ray room
  Basic Radiological System 139, 140
  control unit 123
  daily maintenance 125–126
  monthly maintenance 128
  six-monthly maintenance 129–130
  twelve-monthly maintenance 132
  weekly maintenance 127–128
X-ray tube 121–122
  alignment 129–130
  Basic Radiological System 138
  rotation 130
  spare 143
  stand/support/column 122
X-ray units
  Basic Radiological System specifications 137–138
  control unit 123
  mobile/ward 127
X-rays
  production and use 121
  protection devices 124, 138

www.ingramcontent.com/pod-product-compliance
Ingram Content Group UK Ltd.
Pitfield, Milton Keynes, MK11 3LW, UK
UKHW051524180426
11947UKWH00018B/1562